# WIRED TO HEAL

## RELIEVE STRESS, GET OUT OF YOUR OWN WAY, STAND TALL AND EAT CLEAN

## CASON LEHMAN

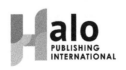

Halo
PUBLISHING
INTERNATIONAL

ISBN: 978-1-63765-029-5
LCCN: 2021908637

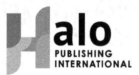

Halo Publishing International, LLC
8000 W Interstate 10, Suite 600
San Antonio, Texas 78230
*www.halopublishing.com*

Printed and bound in the United States of America

For the reader's convenience, and to dig
even deeper into the content of this book,
we have created a resource page for you.

Enjoy!

www.casonlehman.com/wth

# Contents

# Preface

The information I have gathered for this book stems from my calling and my purpose here on this earth. My truth happened to come out through these words, so I simply kept writing. It is my desire to learn more about the human being and our existence on the planet. I have gathered this information through following my heart.

Living a life of chronic pain is not normal. The human being does not just break down like an old car with age. This is a story we have been told. And we believe it.

In fact, regeneration is normal and our bodies are doing it on a moment-to-moment basis. If they were not, you would not be reading this right now. Health and vitality are normal and this is our natural state. Waking up in the morning with great energy, no pain anywhere in our body and a clear, inspired mind is normal. We have just accepted and have been taught that pain and disease are a part of normal aging. We have been conditioned to believe this. We have become programmed. Most of this is not our conscious decision. Most of this programming is below our conscious awareness.

This book will teach you how to stop living as the diagnosis of your disease and to start living as the creation of your desire. When you have worked your way through this book and followed at least most of the advice, you will have arrived at two good places. First, you will have reduced the pain and discomfort that influence your day-to-day life so negatively. Secondly, you will feel better about yourself and in consequence about those around you. You will, in brief, begin to realize that life is beautiful, something to cherish, but like everything else in life that is worth something, you need to put effort into it.

Mom, thank you for showing me what unconditional love was before I even knew. Dad, thanks for believing in my greatness and expecting it. Abbey, thanks for being my biggest supporter and always taking care of me. Also, my editor Frank, for without you popping into my life, this book may not have ever happened. Your wisdom amazes me, and you have been a tower of patience with a sometimes-confused writer.

I dedicate this book to my miracle daughter, Cutler. This, Cutler, is for you and your generation, which I am optimistic will be more aware of their environment and their health than mine has been. For it was not until you manifested into my life that I began to question the current paradigms we live by. I love you, Cutler! But most of all I thank my wife, Chancey, without whose love and constant encouragement I could not have written this book. You, Chancey, are my guiding light and thank you for always bringing me back on track! You show me how to be grateful for the love of life. Thank you all with all my heart.

# Introduction

In my 10 years of practice in physical therapy, I estimate that I have seen more than 10,000 patients with upwards of 20,000 treatments. In nearly all these 20,000 treatments, I am one-on-one with the patient for an entire hour. The patient and I develop a very trusting rapport during their time in Physical Therapy, and I have been able to methodically gather quite a bit of meaningful similarities from my patients.

During this quality time with the patient, I have come to realize that most patients I treat have no clue they alone hold the power to heal their disease. The majority have forgotten the magnificence that lies within. They are unaware of this magnificence, and unbeknownst to them, they are actually the ones who have the primary role in the process of healing their disease. They do not realize they are completely giving their own healing power away, laboring as they are under an illusion that someone or something outside of themselves will heal their dysfunction. They are unaware that they have been conditioned to believe there is a quick fix to their problems, and they just need to find the outside somebody or something that will fix them. Every day I work with patients that have given all their innate healing energy to something outside of themselves only to find out they still have the disease and pain with which they began. On a daily basis I hear things like, "Oh, this is just what happens when you get old." Or "This is just something that

I live with." Or "I've forgotten that I have pain because it's there all the time." My patients think this is perfectly normal, but this is not normal. Otherwise, they would not be searching for an answer by seeing me. We have to acknowledge the fact that we have been conditioned by a society that wants us to believe the answer is from something outside of us that will fix something on the inside of us. Unbeknownst to most people, their biggest opponent is themselves, not the disease.

These material things such as pharmaceutical drugs and surgeries are merely treating the symptoms, further masking the root of the disease. The truth is that pharmaceuticals do not heal chronic conditions. These medications are just merely sustaining a chemical balance in the cell. Pharmaceutical drugs are palliative. Likewise, orthopedic surgeries do not fix or cure the problem either. They are a huge bandage covering up and surgically masking the underlying root cause. Our problem is not the disease or the diagnosis that we have been given—our problem is that we believe we are this thing. Many times, the diagnosis becomes our identity and thus we become a victim to it.

Do not get me wrong, our current medical model has gotten really good at emergency medicine and saving lives. If you break your arm or have appendicitis, you need to see an emergency physician, no doubt. We have prolonged our average life span because of this. But we are lying to ourselves if we do not take into account the quality of our lives. The number of people living in pain, stress and disease is at an all-time high, and it has become an epidemic.

Chronic disease can be defined as conditions that last one year or more and require ongoing medical attention, limit activities of daily living, or both. In 1940, chronic disease prevalence in America was experienced by 7.5% of the population. In 2020, chronic disease was experienced by 60% of the population. And this is just the recorded cases. Think of all the people living in pain and disease that do not go to the doctor. This is a chronic problem, and now is the time to start funneling our resources into the prevention of this epidemic.

Back pain is so common in the United States that it is the second most popular reason people visit their general practitioner.[1] In addition, knee replacements have become common. America does more spine surgeries than anywhere else in the world. In fact, a study all the way back in 1994 found that America does 40% more spine surgeries than the rest of the world and five times more than England and Scotland.[2]

"Total knee replacement utilization in the United States more than doubled from 1999 to 2008." Although the reasons for this increase have not been examined rigorously, some have attributed the increase to population growth and the obesity epidemic[3].

The common pattern I find in all my patients dealing with chronic pain and disease is that they are giving their power away—the power that is the vital life force energy, which is making their very own heartbeat. Just think about it. Who or what is making your heart beat right now as you are reading this? This power is beyond us; it is greater than us. This power can be harnessed and turned inwards and will heal us. The last person believed capable of fixing our own problem is ourselves. All our energy and attention is going to someone (doctor) or something (surgery or pill) to fix us. In order to heal chronic diseases and pain, we must change our lifestyle. We must change our behaviors, make better choices, and learn how to manage our stress.

We must become radically responsible for our own health.

By giving our attention and therefore energy to someone or something outside of ourselves to fix our pain and disease, we are in turn losing precious energy available for the intelligence of our body to utilize for building and repair. Because our medical model primarily uses palliative care to treat symptoms, the patient stays stuck in their disease and pain. We are just simply patching a few holes of the many, and there is no resolution. This becomes a vicious cycle. Not to mention when a health care practitioner, to whom they entrust their lives, tells them their pain or disease is irreversible, and the only prognosis is that it will get worse as the downward spiral continues to exacerbate. A medical professional is a very highly respected member of our society, even more so when there is a Dr. in front of their name. Because of this high regard of respect, the patient takes what the medical professional says as truth; accepting, believing and finally surrendering to whatever they are told.

Let us use the example of chronic low back pain. A person may receive cortisone injections for pain management, giving the patient one day to three months of a pain free life if it works for them. (I hear from my patients many times that the cortisone injection did not create any relief.) This person goes back to the things she loves without any pain. After a certain amount of time, the patient starts to slowly feel the pain creep back into her lower spine. And four months after the injection, the person is experiencing the same amount of pain as before. The patient, still perplexed, and not knowing there is anything else to do for herself, returns to the doctor, believing he is going to fix her. Doc now orders an MRI to get a closer look at what is physically going on in the spine. After looking at the MRI, the doctor tells this patient that he must refer her to a neurosurgeon for there is nothing else he can do.

Respecting this doctor's decision and still being unaware that the fix will actually come from inside of herself, the patient goes to see the surgeon. The surgeon says the only treatment for this condition is a minor back surgery called a laminectomy. The patient's pain is so bad that she agrees because she trusts this surgeon as a professional. The patient undergoes the surgery and has no pain for three years—except the minor discomfort the actual surgery caused, which was very well controlled by narcotic pain medications. One day when this patient bends down to pick up a light box from the floor, she experiences a slightly sharp pain in her back. Over the next couple days, the pain in her low back returns.

Again, this patient is perplexed and does not understand why this pain returned as she was told that the laminectomy would fix the problem. Still, unaware that she has the untapped power within to create a forever fix, she calls the doctor for an appointment to see what is going on. The doctor does not give her any explanation as to why this pain has returned since the visitation is very short, but the doctor does order another MRI to see what is going on in the soft tissues of the spine. The MRI comes back showing no conclusive deformations, so the doctor injects another cortisone shot into her problematic spine, hoping this will relieve some of her pain. This time the cortisone shot does not relieve any pain, and the patient is left baffled again.

This patient is seriously stressed, and the pain is really affecting her life. By chance, the patient sees an ad in the paper for spinal decompression—get rid of back pain with no surgery. She jumps on it! She thinks, "This is it—my fix. This has got to help."

After three weeks of spinal decompression, three times a week the patient has much less pain, however the pain is still not completely gone. When the patient reaches down to pull the trash bag out of the bin, she experiences again the extreme pain in her back, but now the pain is on the other side.

This story could go on and on, and it does for many people living with all sorts of joint pain. I see these patients every single day in my practice. But this story is not just limited to physical pain in the body. It is also a story very similar to patients battling many of the chronic diseases that affect so many lives in America. What this story portrays is what I have heard many call the medical maze. A patient running from specialist to specialist dramatically trying to find the person, pill or machine that will "fix" the problem, yet having seen all these experts, the patient is still left with disease and no relief.

Of the whole, only a very small percentage of medical professionals are empowering the patient to look within themselves for the answer. We have been so conditioned by our schooling, society and the medical system that we, as health care professionals, are meant to fix the patient. The underlying message being taught is we are the expert and the patients are the lay persons. Therefore, the answer comes from us. We believe it is our responsibility to fix them, and equally, they believe we are the person responsible for fixing them. We do not learn anything about the innate power within each of us that has the ability to heal and regenerate from the inside out. Much of the responsibility is dispersed away from the person with the disease.

I feel that a reasonable picture of health for a human being is to have no need for prescription medications for any bodily dysfunction nor a need for any spine operation or joint replacement surgery because of joint pain and dysfunction. Would you not agree that as a society, our goal and mission should be to have fewer replacement surgeries, spine operations, and be prescribed fewer pharmaceutical drugs? To me this is very logical. On the contrary, however, we are now prescribed more pills and endure more orthopedic surgeries than ever before. It would make sense then to direct more of our attention, therefore our energy, into prevention of these diseases and not into the management of the symptoms.

It seems that the polar opposite of this is happening, though, in main stream medicine. I see much more financial, political and educational support being given to palliative care. One of the main reasons this happens is because preventing disease is not billable, therefore, not profitable. Material objects such as medication, surgical tools/parts, medical supplies, and even post-surgical needs such as Physical Therapy all have a price tag. Whereas, preventing something from happening or ever coming back does not. When the patient is empowered, they can choose not to become a victim of the system instead of relying on it in a state of fear.

Fear is a powerful tool, strategically disseminated into the mainstream media by very powerful decision makers to better influence the population's choices. This creates a belief in something that may not have the best interest for the individual. For example, we see it strongly in pharmaceutical advertisements, as at the end of the advertisement, the long list of side effects from the medication are read in fast forward, usually ending with "and may cause death." This is very unfortunate because it shrinks the innate healing power within us all. Fear is now controlling many of our decisions, and when it does, the belief in ourselves fades from our awareness.

Again, to be transparent, there is a time when a joint replacement or emergency back operation is the best option available for the given situation. Likewise, a pharmaceutical drug being used as a treatment for symptom relief and quality of life. However, the use of these alone must be questioned and addressed in an honest conversation.

In this book I will teach you four pillars of knowledge to give back your power forever to fix pain and disease in your body.

The first pillar is stress and how chronic stress creates disease. We will discuss how the majority in our country lives most of their lives in a stressed-out state. You will be able to understand what stress actually is. And you will learn how the hormones of stress cause tissue breakdown in the body leading to pain and disease.

In the second pillar, you will finally understand how to get rid of stress in your life. By having a solid grasp of stress, you will then be better equipped to find where stress is controlling your life. You will be guided through a formula that Joe Dispenza has created, revealing how to become more aware of how you are actually living and being as a human in your day-to-day life. After understanding what masks you are wearing, you will then learn how to create the life of your dreams and bring that life into reality. Then you will learn what meditation is and how to do it. Wait just a second before you say I cannot meditate—I will show you that you can. It is simple and a most effective practice to change your life in an extremely progressive way.

The third pillar is posture. In this section, we will examine in detail how proper posture prevents pain and joint disfunction, as well as how posture can regenerate and heal existing joint pain and dysfunction. You will understand how posture is important to all cellular health and vitality as well as to brain function. You will learn the importance of cerebral spinal fluid and how it and proper posture increase brain function and neuroplasticity.

In this section, you will also learn about how proper posture is directly connected to the hormonal centers of our bodies, what the yogis call the chakras. You will learn where and what each energy center is along our body's central channel and how to use posture combined with your own awareness of these centers to improve the cellular function of each.

The fourth and final pillar of this book examines nutrition. You will realize how on the one hand proper nutrition is essential for the health and repair of our body, while, on the other, processed food and the fast-paced food lifestyle we live in negatively affects our health by contributing to pain and disease. Finally, you will be introduced to the benefits of intermittent fasting and ways to determine if such fasting is right for you. You will also examine the body's circadian rhythms and how the first three pillars tie into the coherence of these rhythms.

## My Story of Transformation

Something was just not right. I was in my late 20s, working at one of the most prestigious outpatient physical therapy clinics in South Florida, absorbing as much knowledge as I possibly could. I was extremely fortunate to land a job working with some of the most decorated fellows of Orthopedic Manual Physical Therapy, and I had just gotten married to the love of my life. My life was really starting to come together. But this did not stop the constant physical and mental pain I was experiencing. I had wandering pain all over my body, my brain was not working properly and my stomach and bowels were always in a knot. Having a bowel movement was extremely painful. I could not go a whole week without asking one of my colleagues to help me out with my wandering orthopedic pain. I would come home after a day of work and pass out in the recliner with exhaustion. I often had to lay down on one of our treatment tables in the clinic at lunch because of fatigue in the middle of the day. I was overweight and could not last more than three weeks on one of those calorie-restricting diets. I exercised all the time, but nothing was working. I mean, I was a high-level athlete previously in my life. Shouldn't I be in great shape? How could I be gaining weight so quickly in my 20s? What was going on? I was dumbfounded.

One of my colleagues, upon new patients' post operation evaluation, would always tell them to stay away from red meat, dairy and shell fish as this can increase the systemic inflammation in their body. This fascinated my curiosity.

"Why is he talking about food after a surgery?" I thought to myself. "What in the world does food have to do with Physical Therapy?"

I always bugged him about why he would say this to the patients, and always being too busy and wanting to talk about sports, he would say, "Oh they just increase inflammation" and shrugged me off. I was not settled. Finally, one day, I pegged him down and got him to spill the beans. He told me that these foods have been found to form inflammatory exudates (toxins) after they are digested, and this then attracts prostaglandins which bind on to the toxins. These inflammatory molecules then end up in the blood stream (We will learn how in Section one). My mind was blown. What were all those big words he just used? We were talking about food being a cause of inflammation. This was the furthest thing from what we learned in Physical Therapy Assistant school. All I knew was I wanted to learn more about inflammation at the cellular level. This captivated me.

Time went by, and I still experienced all sorts of crazy rashes, irritable bowel syndrome, brain fog, constant headaches, chronic fatigue, and I could never breathe out of my nose because it was always stuffed up. I was a mess. My brother-in-law came to Florida to visit on one of his college breaks and started telling me about this new coffee he was drinking that was anti-inflammatory and increased your brain power.

I was like, "What, no way! Does it work?"

He said, "Yeah, all the online poker players are drinking it to have better focus during their time online. It's called Bulletproof Coffee. You should check this guy's website out. He has got tons of great information on there."

Again, this sparked my curiosity as my brother-in-law is very smart. I mean, he had just read an entire book on the plane ride to Florida. I thought to myself, "Who reads books for fun? Wow, he's in college, and he's reading books that his professors did not assign." I never experienced the possibility that you can learn whatever you want to at any time. I was too trapped in the program of keeping up with the Jones's.

Reading from the website, I was blown away. This guy, Dave Asprey, claims that food is the cause of inflammation, pain and disease in our bodies. I thought to myself, "Gee. That's just what my colleague at work is saying about the foods he tells his patients to stay away from." Asprey claims he lost 100 pounds with this lifestyle. I read as many blogs as I could that night, and then I saw that Asprey had a book coming out. So, of course, I bought the book and willed my way through it as I had a very hard time concentrating because of my brain fog. Reading a book was the last thing on my list, but this caught my attention, and my brother-in-law reads, so I thought I should try it out.

I followed the guidelines of the Bulletproof Diet and drank Bulletproof Coffee with grass fed butter and MCT oil blended into it every morning. Two months later I had lost 30 pounds—maybe even more. I do not remember, but all I know is I could start to see some definition in my abs. I never thought I would see that day. This was incredible. I was obviously hooked. Oh, I should mention, in the same time during this lifestyle change, I never felt hungry (well maybe a little bit in the first week, but nothing I could not be greater than), my mind was much sharper, I felt smarter, and I was not falling asleep in the recliner after work. I had so much energy I cooked dinner.

In this lifestyle, I eliminated wheat (gluten), sugar, dairy, corn and soy. This in combination with a drastic increase in consumption of cruciferous vegetables (broccoli, cauliflower, cabbage, Brussels sprouts, kale, etc.) as well as intermittent fasting with Bulletproof coffee, I learned later, is why I started to feel like myself again. We will learn in great detail why all the aforementioned can help you in Section four.

After three or four months of living this way, I had lost 60 pounds, and I felt better than I had ever felt in my life. I was literally in a new body. My irritable bowels had calmed down, and I was able to go to the bathroom pain free for the first time in years. My brain fog was gone, and I felt smarter than I ever had before. So, after I finished the book, I was awakened to a whole new world of other books. This was it! I was committed for life!

But after a year or so went by, I noticed that I was still experiencing random joint pain sometimes. It moved around from my low back, to my shoulder blades, to my neck. I knew this meant I was still inflamed. But how? I was eating the perfect diet. I mean, I lost 60 pounds, what gives? During the previous year or so after I had the dramatic weight loss because of my brain coming back online, I started reading as many books and listening to as many podcasts as I could get my hands on. I had to know more about how nutrition works. And in this pursuit, there was one thing all these books and podcasts always seemed to mention. Meditation. They would always talk about stress running in the background. Mostly, it was discussion about stress caused by food, but nevertheless, stress was always on the docket.

Well, I had to dive into stress and find out what it was about it that created so many problems. I downloaded the calm app and meditated for 10 minutes every morning before work. It felt fantastic but sure enough, random pain would still come back and this left me discouraged. I was not satisfied and it sparked a fire inside to find the answer.

About three years ago, I came across a podcast with a fellow named Joe Dispenza. I decided to watch the video of this podcast, and it blew my mind. It was a bizarre experience that in while listening, I had a very hard time following the complexities of what Dispenza was talking about. At the same time, I was drawn to it like a bug to a light. It spoke to my soul, not my mind. I had to listen three times to better comprehend the philosophical aspect of it, but the same soulful sensation kept burning. So, like I do, I dug deep into his work and continued digging ever since.

It was the pivotal moment of watching that podcast video that tipped the scale of my life from one of victim of my reality to the creator of my reality. I realized I was using food as a scapegoat, not dealing with the underlying shadows of my subconscious that were the real disruptor of my health. The pursuit of knowledge, meditation, postural awareness, and proper nutrition all began to synchronize and created an awakening in my life. It opened the flood gates of my soul, and I could not do anything but listen to what it was telling me. I started becoming more spiritual and studied the mysticism that all the religions talk about. I began to find purpose in my life. I again felt a connection to God and remembered the feeling of a love for life. I started to see the connection of the Divine in nature and learned how there is actually a geometry to the material world. I realized I am the same as everyone else, and no one is better or worse than anyone. All of this has led me to love who I am becoming.

# Section One. New Science:

# Introductory Notions

## All things are possible

Before we jump directly into learning about stress, I want to introduce you to four very important and cutting-edge fields of science that I will be using throughout the book to explain how the four pillars truly work to heal and regenerate your body. The knowledge of these sciences will give us a foundation to catapult our understanding of how to heal our pain and disease. In order to truly make a change, we must have a rooted understanding of how the change will take place. To do so, we must acquire knowledge, and to gain knowledge is to learn. Learning is the basis of our evolution as human beings. Once we learn new information, we become aware of what we were once unaware. When we learn something novel, neurologically, we are creating new neural connections in our brain. These new neural connections create more awareness in our mind. Awareness is consciousness and consciousness is energy. That increase of consciousness is intertwined with an increase of energy in our body. Now we have a memory of which we have learned, and this creates a wonderful feeling within our body. Our brain loves to learn new information, and the whole mind and body process creates a desire for novelties. We are designed to gain knowledge, for this is how we evolved and survived as a species.

Now we have an increase in energy from the excitement of learning something new, and we can use this new information we have acquired and act on it. In other words, we can create a new experience with it. You might call this excitement and enthusiasm inspiration. It is brand new, and thus the novelty inspires us to action. So, we start to practice it because we are inspired to do so. As we repeat this action, it becomes second nature. It becomes a behavior, habit or a skill.

To make the whole learning process more understandable, let us use a simple example of learning to tie your shoe. You first were taught the steps to tie your shoe (novelty), then you practiced tying your shoe repeatedly (action) until finally you could tie your shoe without putting any conscious thought into it (skill). This is where philosophy becomes mastery.

While learning the blueprint for change in this book, I ask that you please maintain an open mind. These new understandings will challenge old belief systems that are currently running our subconscious program about reality. When our old beliefs are challenged with something new and different that does not fit the old model of thinking, our ego tends to cause a bit of chaos in our mind and body. This is because the ego does not like change or the unknown. The ego loves the familiar because it is safe and very predictable. Our ego loves the ability to predict because it already knows what the outcome will be, ensuring safety. This is why changing a habit we know we should change but cannot seem to stop is so hard.

Having a better understanding of the sciences ahead build the neural networks in your brain so you can build a model in your mind to create change in your life.

## Quantum Physics

The first field of science I will explain is Quantum physics. This science is delightfully surprising; it completely challenges our view of reality and turns what we thought we knew upside-down. It is the science that looks at the smallest particles of matter, particularly the atom and the even smaller photon, as well as everything we cannot see yet surrounds us at all times.

In the conventional model of Newtonian Physics, we view ourselves as solid, stable and most of all separate things. Most of our modern thoughts are based on our physical universe being made up of things. These things are in turn made up of teenier things. In order to understand the bigger material things, we must better understand the smaller things. This creates a belief that things made up of littler things are separate from us.

The study of Newtonian physics is based on our three-dimensional world and everything in it. It is based on materialism. Thanks to Newtonian physics, we can figure out how long it will take us to travel from point A to point B. Point A and point B are separate and have their own locality. If we know what forces are acting on a material object, then we can determine its exact position and velocity at any given time. In essence, Newtonian physics is all about predictability.

You probably remember the Styrofoam ball and toothpick model of the atom from your high school science class (Niels Bohr illustrative model), where there was a central nucleus made up of protons and neutrons, and then electron molecules were orbiting around the nucleus in very predictable order—like the earth orbits around the sun. We were taught that this atom was a fixed molecule that, when combined with more atoms, makes up the things in our physical world, like the chair you are sitting on and the book you're reading. The concept of all material things being made up of atoms seems to be correct. However, when quantum scientists such as Werner Heisenberg took a closer look at the atom, things got pretty strange.

Things started to act in a very unpredictable way. When Heisenberg and his colleagues looked at the smallest particles of matter, they found something very weird that we now know as *the uncertainty principle*. They found that when their conscious attention (directed energy) was on the atom it turned into matter or *something*, but when they took their attention off the atom or particle, it turned into *nothing*. The *nothing* was the electron, and it turned into an electron cloud of possibility. It was not a fixed, predictable thing.

This, in quantum physics, is known as the wave function. So only through the act of a person observing the atom did it manifest into something material. When the observer was not looking at the object, it turned into the unknown or potential. Quantum physics has now named this *the observer effect*. It is a bit mind-blowing because when the observer (the scientist) has his attention directed on an object (he or she is looking at it), it turns into matter. But when the observer takes his or her attention off the perceived thing, it turns into nothing. This nothing is actually not nothing, it is just invisible to the human eye. It is essentially a wave of energetic possibility.

According to Heisenberg's uncertainty principle, we now understand that an electron cloud floats around the atom. This electron cloud has infinite potential, meaning we never know where the electron will be, and it literally has the potential energy to turn nothing into something. In other words, it turns the unknown into the known. This new understanding took all the previous Newtonian physics principles and threw them out the window.

To better understand these phenomena, let us consider what lives in the invisible space all around us. Through our five senses (sight, smell, taste, touch and hearing), we perceive the world around us as separate and disconnected (people, places and things). But when we take a closer look, we find a vast inexhaustible energy source sitting untouched in the space around us. This energy surrounding us carries information and has infinite potential. This is known as the field. And all possibilities exist in the field.

In order to better comprehend this energy field, let us take a look at the visible spectrum of light compared to the light we cannot see. This light is always around us in our three-dimensional world. In other words, let's look at what we can see with our eyes, compared to what we cannot see with our eyes. (Remember, all light is energy, and all energy carries a specific frequency or vibration.) We do not pay attention to this field of energy available to us at all times because we cannot see it or always feel it with our senses. However, all this light (energy) carries billions and billions of tiny bits of information, always around us and accessible at every moment.

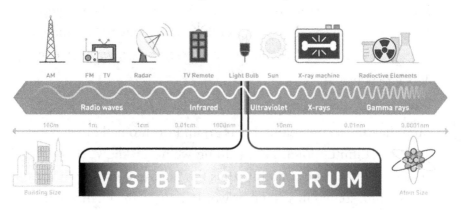

*Figure 1-As the light spectrum moves toward the right of the diagram the frequency increases, coming closer to zero-point energy. As it moves left, it becomes denser as the frequency slows. We are only able to perceive with our eyes a small fraction of the entire spectrum, shown here as the visible spectrum. The visible spectrum are the colors of the rainbow.*

Our eyes can only perceive less than 1% of the light (energy) that exists. In the diagram above, when we look at the light spectrum of electromagnetic frequencies, we can see the visible light is only a small fraction of what exists. We see that the higher the frequency, the closer the light gets to the zero-point field, and the other end of the spectrum is a much slower frequency which is becoming more matter or density. This makes sense because as energy slows down or becomes a slower frequency, it becomes denser. Think of all matter as compressed, dense energy.

Water and its different states are a perfect example of how matter becomes more or less dense based on its frequency. As water's frequency slows, it becomes denser and turns to ice. Conversely, as its frequency speeds up, it becomes less dense and lighter and then turns into steam first and then into vapor. Similarly, when you pack a snowball, you are creating an object (ball) with more density.

Now let us look at an everyday example to better help us comprehend the invisible field of energy around us by taking a moment to think about your car radio. You can hear the music playing from your speakers, and you can tune in to a number of different radio stations, but you cannot see the connection. An invisible radio wave in the field matches a certain radio station which is playing using its own frequency. When the frequency of the transducer in your car radio matches the frequency of the station coming from the radio tower transmitting it, there is a vibrational match. Because of this vibrational match, sound is manifested through our speakers. Magic! This information always surrounds us and, in this case, is being picked up by our car radio and turned to music.

In order to truly transform your life into your dream, it is essential to understand this. Just because you cannot see something does not mean it does not exist. When you comprehend this state neurologically through learning the principles of quantum physics, you now open the doors of possibilities. Personally, there is nothing more inspiring than new possibilities.

Side note: We actually see with our brain. Our eyes pick up light (energy) from the field all around us. This light is filled with information. The eyes send this information through the optic nerve to the visual cortex in our brain. The visual cortex of the brain processes this information into imagery. We are constantly picking up frequencies or information in wave forms that create patterns and turning that information into imagery in our minds. This is a quantum phenomenon.

Another piece of the quantum physics study we must understand to better heal ourselves and create the life of our dreams are the theories of locality versus non-locality. In Newtonian physics, locality is understood to mean that you cannot interact with something separate from you without sending some kind of signal to it. This signal needs transmission through the space between you and that thing. The important understanding from this is that it was believed all signals take time to travel from one thing to another separate thing. And this would mean, based on the conventional understanding, that there is an upper limit to the speed of how fast things can travel. This is what Einstein believed to be the speed of light.

Non-locality means no separation—that all things are connected. In quantum entanglement, scientists have found that two separate photons (a light particle smaller than an atom) simultaneously are entangled. This means that when an action is performed on one, it simultaneously is done on the other even when these tiny light particles are separated great distances. Einstein called this phenomenon "spooky action at a distance" as he still believed that the speed of light was the fastest speed possible. We now know this to be untrue as these separate particles act as one. This means they are not separate.

From this invisible field of information comes everything that exists. Albert Einstein said that the field is the sole governing agency of the particle (matter). Let us think about this based on the quantum model of reality. This would mean that an invisible field of energy connects all things (everybody, everyone, everything and everywhere) beyond space and time. When we break down things into the smallest subatomic particles, we see that nothing except possibility exists. So, this must mean a governing consciousness creates this potential into matter.

Everything is connected invisibly through energy in the field, and all this invisible energy carries information. The fact is there is really no such thing as objects, as science has not been able to compartmentalize matter into anything definitive. You and everything around you are a collection of charged energy having a relationship. The closer scientists look, the more they find that everything is dependent on and indivisible from everything else. When they get down to the bottom layer of matter, they find a little puff of nothingness that somehow coalesces with the governing field of energy, all based on where we place our attention. These little puffs of energy are in fact just potential that can be affected by us, which Heisenberg proved with the uncertainty principle. In fact, it is something. It actually is everything, but it yet has been manifested into what we can see. It is the source from which everything physical is created.

This is mind-blowing, I know. But in truth, science cannot prove whether the smallest particles we can break matter down to are actually a particle or a wave of possibility that turns into a particle. Many experiments are being done to find the mathematics behind what is true. Constantly trying to prove and disprove what makes our three-dimensional world. The important take away is this—the observer has an influence on matter, making it appear or disappear. I would say that means we have some serious, powerful capabilities when our intentions are clear.

One tangible example of the field and the invisible connection between all things that we can all relate to are synchronistic events. We might have taken for granted that these events may have been random coincidences, but are they?

Think of the times when you have picked up your phone to call a friend or a family member, and just as you pick the phone up to dial their number, the phone rings and it is that exact person you were going to call. Or when you have been thinking of any random object and you drive past a billboard with that symbol on it. We think all of this is coincidence, but science is beginning to help us understand why this happens. We are all connected to one larger whole of which we are made by way of our cells, but we do not believe it because we cannot see it. Remember—just because you cannot see it does not mean it does not exist. We now use Bluetooth and Wi-Fi every day in most all our daily lives. We cannot see what it is that is allowing our cell phone to connect to the Internet to check our Instagram, yet we use it and rely on it all day long.

We have been conditioned to being separate from everyone, everything and everywhere, but the truth is we are all connected to a much greater governing consciousness. This is so exciting because what this means is we literally create our own reality. We are the observer, and we have the ability to be aware that we are aware. Life does not happen to us—it actually happens through our perception of it. This means we can be greater than our outside world. Our reality is manifested by who we are being. Our state of being. This is the way we think, the way we feel and the way we behave. Because we have the free will to change all those things, this means we have the power to create the life we want. We will take an in-depth look into how this happens based on our state of being in section two: how to get out of stress and create lasting change in our life.

## Photons

The second branch of science that will help in our understanding of how to unleash our incredible untapped potential is a new science that looks at the smallest form of light (energy) called a photon.

In 1996, a German scientist Fritz Albert Popp founded the International Institute of Biophysics (IIB). In his work, Popp discovered biophotons, tiny low-intensity light particles stored within and emitted by all living things. These photons are high frequency light-energy particles. Remember from the above that light is energy and all things emit light. Popp and his researchers believed that these tiny light particles, which are stored in DNA, communicates extremely effectively with the cells of the organism, thus playing a vital role in regulating the function of the organism.

The photon is so small it is considered to have no mass. It is the bridge between a particle and energy, and it also acts in that way. When scientists test to see if it is a physical mass, it tests as though it is. When it is tested to see if it is quantum energy, it acts as energy. It has the ability to respond to our thoughts and expectations. When scientists study an observer's attention, they find that where the observer places his attention increases the photon density of that object. This helps us construct a model in our mind of how the observer effect works. The mind's attention or awareness on something literally rearranges the photon density in accordance with that focused attention. This means where we focus our attention and therefore energy literally affects stuff in the material world.

The study of photons proves that the cells of our body communicate most effectively through electromagnetic energy (light). Inside each of our cells we have tiny skeletal particles called microtubules and these tuning fork-like tissues are able to pick up the frequencies of vibration or light energy in a faster way than chemical interchange between the cells. These impulses communicated by photons send information faster than the synapses of neurons in our nervous system. This happens at a quantum level and is how our cellular biology functions. In doing so, they exchange vital information, and when the cells energy and frequencies are more coherent or organized, the better the cell functions. Popp found that the opposite is also true—namely that when a cell is emitting a lower coherent and unorganized electromagnetic field, it functions less optimally and becomes unhealthy.

To give an example, imagine a group of five-year-old children whom each have access to their own drum, and they are all beating on their drums in an incoherent, random and erratic fashion. This would be torturous to our ears. This is similar to how our cells are systemically functioning in a disease and pain state in our body. Now, imagine a college marching band's drumline creating rhythmic, inspiring beats with their coherent and organized cadence. This makes the hair on the back of your neck stand up in an amazing way. This is analogous to the coherence and order in a healthy body's state. This rhythm is what we will learn to induce in the cells of our body throughout this book.

Popp's study has huge implications, because this means the biochemical model we learned in high school is dated. Popp discovered that the electromagnetic energy the cell emits is the primary mode of function for the cell's life and health. This energy is what controls those molecules of biochemistry. All biochemistry of the cell follows an energy or a frequency because all matter is an energy or vibration.

To understand that we are energetic beings, let us break it down this way. Subatomic particles (photons) make up an atom. A large group of atoms make up a molecule. A group of specific molecules make up a chemical. A group of specific chemicals make up a cell, a group of cells make up a tissue, a group of tissues make up an organ, a group of organs make up an organ system, and a group of systems make up the human organism. So then, when we look closely at what we are actually made of, we find we are merely just energy.

The human being is an astonishing and miraculous machine of functions we take for granted every second of every day. And when we lack the circuitry of coherent and rhythmic energy, therefore causing the cell not to function in its most optimal way, we, as a whole unit, do not function as we should. This causes a group of cells to function improperly with decreased energy, which causes the tissue to break down, which then causes the organ to function less orderly. Then cascading to the system, we have a full-blown disease. Thus, to reverse our pain and disease, it would make sense that we must increase the coherent energy within our body.

## Psychoneuroimmunology

Now that we understand how much power we have over our reality, let us look at the emerging field of science called *Psychoneuroimmunology*. This new science will help us broaden our understanding of how we can heal ourselves. You have probably heard the phrase *mind over matter*. This is the science that explains how that well-known phenomena happens. The definition of psychoneuroimmunology is the study of the effect of the mind on health and resistance to disease. By now I hope you are awakened to the fact that this is a real thing, so let us break this science down a little further.

The moment we have a thought in our mind, the brain secretes and releases neurotransmitters. A neurotransmitter is a chemical substance that is released at the end of a nerve fiber to create a synapse or a connection with another nerve cell in our brain. Every thought has thousands of the synaptic connections firing all day long. With each of these synapses, a specific and unique chemical concoction of neurotransmitters is being released. The signature of these neurotransmitters then has a cascade effect on the more automatic part of our brain called the limbic brain. The limbic brain is the part of the brain that controls the automatic functions of our body like our heart rate, respiration rate, blood pressure and body temperature. We will discuss the brain and its functions in more depth in the next chapter.

For now, it is important to understand that the thoughts we think influence another chemical called a neuropeptide. Neuropeptides are made in response to the release of the chemical signature of neurotransmitters. These neuropeptides work their way into the blood stream and transmit messages to the body, influencing the hormonal cells to produce the respective hormones associated with that center. This is the basics of how an emotion is created biochemically. And again, just as photons are the basis of every biochemical reaction process, they are here too. This biochemistry trail we can measure seems to be a footprint left in the material world, while this phenomenon of a thought simultaneously creating an emotion is happening faster than the speed of light. The important take away from all this science is pure and simply that emotions (thoughts and feelings) are turned into chemistry that influences every cell of the body. Which means the way you think and feel has a primary effect on your health.

## Thinking and Feeling, Feeling and Thinking Feedback Loop

This process does not just happen from the brain to the body. It also happens in reverse, where the body influences the brain. When the cells of the body receive these messages from neuropeptides, they are receiving instructions for cellular functions such as what proteins to manufacture in the nucleus of the cell. In time, the cell gets accustomed to these messages based on our attitude or state of being. When we subconsciously live in a certain state like fear, worry, doubt, shame, being a victim or blame, our cells are receiving that chemical cocktail the majority of our days.

As the cell becomes familiar with the fearful state we are living in, it sends messages back to the brain to tell the brain it wants more of those feelings. The brain gives in and consequently has more thoughts in the state of fear, worry, doubt, lack, etc. This creates a feedback loop from thinking to feeling and then feeling to thinking. The brain and the body get stuck in a program. They get stuck in a box in their conscious world that is being driven subconsciously. Living in this fear state program lowers our energy and causes incoherence in the cells, tissues and body.

To broaden our study, let us use an example of a habitual thought with a strong emotion tied to it. Imagine that every night when you lie down in bed, just as you have gotten comfortable, you have a thought of "oh no, did I remember to lock the front door?" You try your hardest to let it go, but the fear of someone being able to walk in unobtrusively through your front door lingers in your mind. You cannot stop thinking about it, so your body tells your mind that it must get up out of your warm and comfortable bed to go and check the front door, making sure you have locked it. What has happened biochemically is you created a specific blend of neurotransmitters based on your thought, that influenced a specific blend of neuropeptides which then make their way into the body and create a feeling of worry. Now you are in the state of worry and fear all based on a thought alone. The body becomes programmed to this state subconsciously and wants more of these chemicals. As much as you want to stay in bed, you cannot because your body has become your mind. This is why you have a hard time just letting this thought go as you are in your warm comfortable bed. The body has been chemically conditioned to this emotion, and it wants it. It knows it. And it tends to identify as it.

## Epigenetics

In order to examine how this process of who we are being (attitude) can either be a catalyst to our health, giving us lasting longevity, or a health disrupter, causing tissue break down and disease, we now must understand a bit about the new science of Epigenetics. Epigenetics literally means above genetics.

We have all been brought up and conditioned to believe the genetics we inherited from our parents and past generations before them will predetermine our life's health. Because of the new science of epigenetics, we now know this is untrue. Epigenetics proves that genes are not a set-in-stone direction for our predetermined destiny. Epigenetics proves we have the ability to influence our genes through environment and lifestyle. This new science proves that the power lives within us.

What is a gene, anyway?

Genes are made in the nucleus of the cell, and they are responsible for the production of proteins. A gene is a sequence of nucleotides that carries a special code based on the combination of four amino acids called, adenine, guanine, cytosine and thiamine. The combination of these four amino acids within the nucleotide creates a special code which fabricates all the proteins in our body.

This means that in every cell of our body, a gene carries the code for the production of that specific protein. These proteins then make up our structures (bones) as well as carrying out specific functions (like enzymes as a catalyst for a cellular action) throughout our entire body, with an exception of red blood cells.

(Mature red blood cells do not have a nucleus.) Scientists have found around 140,000 different proteins that are being made over and over again in our body. This means that a different gene code is responsible for making each of these specific proteins. it is important to note that this does not mean we have 140,000 separate genes to make the 140,000 proteins, as we will discuss in a minute.

But first, remember that every cell makes up a tissue and a tissue and organ and so on. Now when we go back to the cellular level and look at how proteins are manufactured in every cell, we see how critically important they are as they make up the entire structure and the function of our body. The word protein comes from the Greek word proteios and proteios means primary. Proteins are primary as they bring our body to life. To give an example of how proteins act in the function of our body, let's look at the digestive system. In the digestive cells of our body, genes are responsible for programming the code to create new enzymes. Enzymes are a protein and their function is to breakdown food by splicing it into its more digestible smaller parts.

To give another example of the importance of proteins, consider a different organ of our body. Consider the muscle cell. In the muscle cell, specific genes are responsible for the creation of new and healthy muscle tissue. This is done by the nucleus of a muscle cell transcribing proteins called actin and myosin. Actin and myosin are responsible for the contraction of our muscles. When a muscle contracts, it moves our body.

These are just two examples of specific proteins in our body. The further magnitude of proper gene expression is vast. Almost infinite. So, you can see the importance of the genetic program that is being either turned on or turned off predominantly by our state of being, to create the structure and function of our body. Quite simply put, our health is directly connected to how well our genes are creating or turning off the production of specific proteins. This is within our control.

As a matter of fact, thanks to the Human Genome Project, we have learned that our genes make more than 140,000 proteins in our body. 40,000 of the 140,000 proteins turn out to be regulatory proteins (proteins that help to make other more complex proteins). These are still essential, nonetheless.

During the Human Genome Project, when scientists took a closer look at the gene itself, they only found 23,688 individual genes. This took the scientists of the Human Genome Project and especially the investors, who were banking on their hypothetical predictions, by a huge surprise. Before the investigation into our genome took place, they predicted that because genes make proteins, there should be a 1:1 ratio of genes to proteins. They hypothesized that because there are 23,688 individual genes there would be 23,688 reciprocal proteins made by each gene. To their surprise, what they found was that one gene has the potential to make hundreds to thousands of different proteins all on its own.

What this finding shows is that the probability of mapping genes can almost have an infinite number of outcomes. Which is impossible for anyone to predict. After further research, we have found that of the entire 100% of what proteins our genes can make, we are only expressing 1.5% of that. This leaves 98.5% of our potential gene expression untouched and unexpressed.

Scientists have labeled the untouched 98.5% junk DNA. This untouched DNA is not junk! This dormant DNA is unlimited potential just waiting to be expressed. We literally have unlimited potential of health, wellness, abundance, love, confidence, manifestation, greatness, etc. available in our genome, sitting untouched. There is nothing more inspirational than this fact alone. Talk about infinite possibilities. We have so much unknown potential just waiting to be switched on right inside every one of our cells.

The question is, what causes a gene to produce one certain protein and not another? And further, how can we unleash that dormant potential in each of us? Can we turn on healthy genes and turn off unhealthy disease-causing genes?

The answer is an absolute, YES!

We can do this by changing the environment around the cell. When we change our attitude (how we think and how we feel), we can absolutely switch on health promoting genes and conversely turn off disease promoting genes. Although the environment outside our body is very important and no doubt has an effect on our genetic expression, the environment inside our body but outside the cell is the most critical.

## Inside Our Body But Outside The Cell

We have learned enough new information about psychoneuroimmunology to understand that our thoughts influence the health of our body. Remember, this happens via neuropeptides being released into the blood from the brain and in turn flowing down into the body to influence the cells of our hormonal centers, causing them to release their specific chemicals into our bloodstream. We now must understand how this influences the gene inside the cell. Another way to understand psychoneuroimmunology and epigenetics is to understand that our state of being or our mood in any moment is directly influencing what genes are being expressed and what genes are not inside the cell's nucleus. Psychoneuroimmunology and epigenetics are divinely synchronized with each other as the cell is constantly receiving neuropeptide signals based on how we think and feel all on a quantum biology level.

In his book *The Biology of Belief*, Bruce Lipton found in his lab that the environment of the cell is the determining agent for which gene is expressed and which repressed. He found that the cell membrane, which he calls the cell memBRAIN, is the intelligence service of the cell constantly receiving and sending information through a lock and key type of mechanism in the membrane of the cell. The cell memBRAIN has thousands of tiny antennas coming from it, endlessly picking up frequencies to which it responds. This finding is very similar to what Popp discovered in his studies of biophotons and the ability of the microtubules to pick up vibrational frequencies. Based on the information the memBRAIN picks up, the cell then either allows neuropeptides, hormones and other messengers to either enter the cell or reject them from entering. This process of neuropeptides, hormones and other messengers being processed by the memBRAIN and then to either be allowed into the cell or not, is what instructs the nucleus to turn the precise gene on or off.

What this means is the cell memBRAIN is picking up the specific chemical vibration based upon our mood or attitude. Our attitude and state of being have a specific chemical signature being released into our bodies at all times. Keep in mind that our energetic vibration is measurable which we'll learn about later in section three. This is based on how we are thinking and feeling and feeling and thinking. To say this another way, your attitude is directly correlated to your health. Who you are being is everything. Your thoughts directly affect the cell by actually turning into the chemical signature that the cell membrane picks up through the vibrational frequency of that specific mood.

As we think and feel, feel and think, the chemical cocktail of our specific thought and feelings are sent into our body, telling the hormonal centers which chemicals to produce. As this chemical cocktail of hormones is released into the blood stream, the signature starts to communicate with all the cells of our body; we are signaling genes to either upregulate or downregulate in the individual cells of the entire body. At a quantum level, signals are sent to the cell like text messages. This is all happening via frequencies the memBRAIN is able to transduce. The cell then responds to this message by sending information to the nucleus of the cell to make a certain protein by way of gene expression.

If we are living by the same thoughts and same feelings every day, we are therefore telling our cells to make the same proteins day in and day out, all by way of the gene production in the nucleus. While living in this same old state of being, it means that the same 1.5% of our genome is repeatedly being expressed again and again. Over time, that gene that is expressed repeatedly becomes weaker, which means a weaker protein. Think about our skin. Our skin is made from proteins, and as we age, the skin becomes looser and less elastic. This is due to the proteins that make our skin becoming worn out and weak after being expressed repeatedly.

Imagine a copy machine. If the copy machine were to make a copy of the copy multiple times, the picture quality would become weaker and more distorted. This is analogous to what happens to the proteins made by our genes when we are living in the same stress daily. The proteins weaken, and we age and become susceptible to disease.

Immune functions are controlled by proteins. When the genes responsible for making these proteins are not being turned on because they have to account for us living in fear, they are not in abundance to take care of foreign invaders or cancer cells. You can see what is left to happen. Disease of some sort.

It only makes sense then to stop wiring and firing those same old thoughts every day which are wearing out the same old 1.5% of genes being expressed, in turn making a weaker protein. By thinking and feeling, and feeling and thinking, in higher states of being, which is the vibration of love, we now can tap into the 98.5% of available potential. By changing our state, we are now tapping into the potential of health, regeneration, healing, new opportunities and better overall function. The 98.5% of the dormant, abundant bank of genetic potential is just waiting for us to turn it on like an enthusiastic athlete waiting to be called in by the coach.

It is clearly obvious that the many centenarians throughout the world are vibrantly healthy at a ripe old age because of this. They are in love with life. They turn a so-called negative situation into a positive learning opportunity in order to grow. They are connected to a higher power. They grow and eat their own food in healthy organic soil that they dig in with their own two hands. They work in the garden with love in their hearts. They get outside and do work they love dearly. They live for themselves and not based on what someone else has told them they should do.

I don't know about you, but I have never met an angry 100-year-old. And now you can see why they have made it 100 plus years on planet earth. They are tapping into the 98.5%!

## Placebo and Nocebo Effect

A placebo is an inert substance like a sugar pill, a saline injection or even a fake surgery that is designed to have no therapeutic value. Scientists use the placebo to compare against the actual substance created in their lab. In a clinical trial, for example, one group of individuals receive the real therapeutic substance, one group a placebo in which they do not know is a placebo but are told is the real drug, and one group called a control group will be given nothing. The scientists then test objective findings such as blood markers as well as subjective reports of how the individuals in the respected groups felt after taking the pill or getting the injection.

The placebo effect *really* does work. In fact, the placebo effect according to Bruce Lipton[4] is responsible for at least one third of all healing in medical interventions. This is not the sugar pill or a saline injection that is doing the healing; it is the patient's belief that is doing the healing. And what does a belief do? It creates a state of being or an attitude, which influences the gene of the cell to produce new proteins in new ways. Now the body—by way of genetic expression—turns on genes to make proteins that perform the healing and regeneration. The body also turns off the genes responsible for the inflammation and thus causes the disruption of the disease. This is all done by thought (belief) processes alone.

What is even more astounding is the nocebo effect. This is the opposite of the placebo effect. If the placebo heals the body, the nocebo can actually kill a person. If following an ankle injury, a patient is told by the doctor he or she can never again run, and the patient accepts, believes and surrenders to this one doctor's medical advice, then the patient will never run again based on a belief. Same thing goes for a terminal diagnosis.

Many very weird and extreme medical events have been documented because of the nocebo effect. A particular reported case happened to a man in the 1970s who was given a terminal diagnosis of cancer and told by the doctor he only had three months to live. Sure enough, the man died in three months. But things got even stranger when the man's autopsy revealed he did not have the type of terminal cancer that he was misdiagnosed with. He had a different type of cancer that the pathologist determined was NOT a terminal diagnosis. This man died from thought alone.[5]

Quite morbid, I know, but the point is for you to understand how powerful our beliefs are. You can see clearly now that we have the power within us to heal. But we also have the power within to make us sick if we become our diagnosis.

All these new sciences lead to possibility. They show us there is much more to learn and understand than what we observe with our five senses. By having an understanding of the "new" science we open our awareness to new possibilities never before in our consciousness. We now have so much information available to us that we can no longer be unconscious of the fact that we are intelligent beings beyond our current perception. Throughout this book, we will learn how to unleash the power within each of us just waiting to be revved up in order for us to heal our pain, reverse our disease and catapult our life to a whole new understanding of love.

## Quick Takeaways of the New Sciences

1. Everything is connected, which means we are connected to our future healing that has not yet happened in our three-dimensional reality.

2. We are made of energy, which is simply vibrations of information.

3. Our thoughts become things and influence the cells of our body.

4. The cells of our body become accustomed (addicted) to our state of being and send messages to the brain to think more of the familiar thoughts.

5. This makes change very difficult.

6. Only 1.5% of the entirety of our genetic material is expressed at any given moment.

7. This means there is 98.5% that sits waiting to be turned on or turned off.

8. Altogether, this means we have a power beyond our comprehension both inside (our cells) and outside (the field) of our body to heal us.

9. What we believe matters. What we accept, believe and surrender to create biochemistry in our body.

# Section Two. Stress:

# Bane of Modern Life

## *Stress or why pain and disease are so common today.*

In this section, we will take an in-depth look at stress. You will learn how stress is secretly running the show in your body and how it goes mostly unnoticed while knocking your body out of its smooth-flowing rhythm of natural health. Chronic stress and its detriment to our body are the first of the four pillars I will teach you in this book. Knowing what stress is, becoming aware of it, and knowing when your body is being unconsciously run by it will have the biggest impact on returning to your innate health. Simply becoming aware of what stress is doing in the background all day long is foundational in change. For you must know the problem in order to fix it. This will give you the power of choice, and it will allow you to take your innate power back.

We will learn what stress actually is and how the hormones of stress lead to tissue breakdown, pain and dis-ease. We will learn about the autonomic nervous system, how it is broken down into two systems—the parasympathetic and sympathetic nervous systems—and how either one or the other regulates our body's automatic functions. We will continue to go more into depth in the field of psychoneuroimmunology and epigenetics and explore how the hormones released from stress called corticosteroids become an addiction to the cells of our body. We will view how stress causes improper digestion of food by stealing the energy away from our gut. Finally, we will learn how the hormones of stress cause us to crave the wrong kind of foods leading to weight gain while creating a negative feedback loop into obesity and systemic inflammation.

In today's medical world, we cannot pinpoint the cause of most all the diseases spiraling out of control in our Western society. Of all dis-ease, only about 1-5% of them are caused because of an actual genetic mutation in the DNA blueprint. These are diseases such as cystic fibrosis, sickle cell anemia, type-1 diabetes, Huntington's disease. When we study pathophysiology and dive into the cause of dis-ease in our medical training, we find "etiology unknown" under most of the common diseases in today's world. In layman's terms, this means we do not know the reason for this dis-ease or, furthermore, its cause. We have become very good at diagnosing dis-ease, though when it comes down to curing and reversing the dis-ease we are left chasing our tails.

So then, why are there so many diseases, but so few solutions? Why do so many people live with pain that keeps coming back after short-lived respite from it? Why are we now sicker and more obese than we have ever been in human history?

I attest that stress and our unconscious awareness of it running the show in our body is the underlying cause of most of our pain and disease today.

Stress is defined as anytime the body gets knocked out of balance. The body's balance is called homeostasis. Stress has been the vital function for our survival as a species. In the course of our evolution, had we not possessed the stress response, we would not have been able to mobilize enough energy to escape lethal threats, and therefore end our time here on earth. During the stress response, the massive amounts of energy our body uses for things like digestion, healing, repair, and growth are blunted to ensure our survival.

When we perceive a threat in our environment, our body automatically transfers energy to increase our heart rate so we can pump more blood and oxygen to our muscles in order to have a better ability to run, fight or hide. Hormones are automatically released into our blood stream to give the body a rush of energy. Our blood and therefore the oxygen supply is also rerouted in large quantities to our brain as compared to what is used in our resting state. This provides us with the ability to heighten our memory recall, making us super-aware, and increases our survival potential in a life-threatening event. The bronchioles in our lungs dilate in order to ventilate our body with fresh oxygen to outrun a predator. The pain receptors in our body are desensitized to allow us to be pain free while we run or fight for survival. Our immune system and blood clotting factor is also temporarily ramped up to ensure any of the wounds we incur during fight or flight can be mended and sanitized from any pathogens.

The stress process is absolutely amazing, and the fact that the body can engage in this without our conscious awareness is even more so, but there is one major problem—the body is not made to stay in this mode for long periods.

In nature, when a gazelle escapes the near fatal attack of a lioness, its body bounces back into homeostasis in a matter of minutes after this stress response. The gazelle, unlike humans, does not replay the event repeatedly in the frontal lobe of its brain. Its frontal lobe is substantially smaller than ours. In fact, the human frontal lobe is much larger than any other animal, giving us the ability of metacognition. Metacognition is our ability to be aware that we are aware. In section two, this subject will be further elaborated, and the reader will learn to master it.

In our over-stimulated, fast paced world today, there is also a disadvantage to this massive frontal lobe, namely that our super-powered brain can continue to remember the stressful event ever so frequently. Let's face it, we are no longer being chased by predators in the wild or having to weather a massive storm without shelter.

Today, our stress is mainly created by thought alone.

Worry, anxiety, guilt and many more fearful emotions are habitually played out in the brain throughout our days.

Things such as the amount of money in our bank account, whether we remembered to lock the front door, the argument we had with our spouse, and the guilt we hold on to for yelling at our children for the mess they make every day continually run through our minds all day long. Every time our mind goes back to the thought of stress, we recreate the experience biochemically in our brain and body. Whereas, the gazelle lets go and simply goes back to grazing. Consequently, the gazelle population does not have a high incidence of stress-related diseases like cancer, multiple sclerosis, eczema, depression, Alzheimer's, obesity, heart disease, arthritis, low-back pain, neck pain, joint pain, diabetes, gastrointestinal dysfunction.

Hopefully you can see the writing on the wall here. If not, let me make it clear—stress is the cause of the majority of pain and disease in our society today. Before we go into detail about how this happens biochemically, let us first go into a little more depth about our autonomic nervous system and the nuts and bolts of the human stress response.

To further understand the stress response and the autonomic nervous system, we must learn some basic information about the brain, the mind and how thought is developed. The brain is far too complex to describe in three layers, but for better understanding and for the purposes of this book, think of the brain in three parts. The neo cortex, the limbic brain and the reptilian brain.

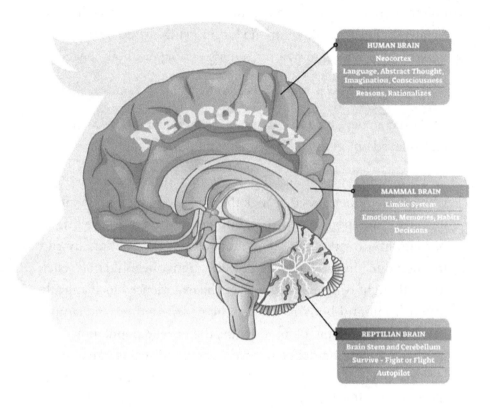

*Figure 2*

The neocortex is the outermost part of the brain and where the folds of our grey matter are housed. In the outer space of our brain, we have the cerebrum which is broken up into two hemispheres—the left and the right. Our right side of the cerebrum is responsible for things such as creativity, imagination, musical skills and artistic skills. The left side of the brain is responsible for things such as math skills, scientific thinking, logical thinking, spoken and written language.

In the grey matter folds of the neocortex are where most of the synaptic connections of our thoughts take place. When the cells of the brain are firing and wiring, this is called the mind. The mind is the brain in action. The mind is how we mysteriously see pictures and images in our consciousness (our mind's eye). It is what we see in the form of images which arise from the synaptic connections from neuron to neuron in a nearly infinite orchestra of daily thoughts. The mind functions in polarity or duality. The mind loves to analyze. It classifies things right or wrong, black or white, good or bad, male or female. We, as the mind, spend the majority of our time analyzing, predicting, assuming and judging every detail of our day. Just as the neocortex has a left and a right side that function in polar opposites, this is exactly how our mind in whole performs best.

The Autonomic Nervous System operates just like its name implies, and it is in charge of the automatic functions of the body. It is responsible for things like our heart beating, our heart rate, blood pressure, body temperature regulation, insulin regulation, and so much more. The autonomic nervous system is split up into two parts—the sympathetic nervous system, which you may have heard of as the "fight-or-flight system" and the parasympathetic nervous system, which is the inverse, known as the "rest and digest" nervous system. The body is run by either one system or the other. I like to break it down into parasympathetic equals love and sympathetic equals fear.

The Autonomic Nervous System functions deeper in the center of our brain, which is home to our limbic and reptilian brain. In these more primitive parts of the brain, our thoughts and feelings become integrated into our body. This is the home of the mind-body connection. When we have a thought, the neuron sends an electrical impulse through its axon arm into its finger-like dendrites to create a synapse with another nerve cell in the brain. This synapse creates a chemical release from nerve cell to nerve cell. This is happening in thousands of nerve cells all at once for every thought going through our brain. This chemical release has a specific and individual chemical signature that the neocortex sends down to the limbic brain. Here again, we see that this firing and wiring is happening at a quantum level beyond our comprehension. No science can yet fully comprehend this phenomenon.

What we do know, however, is that the limbic brain receives this chemical message and creates a molecule called a neuropeptide specific to the signature of the thought in the brain. This neuropeptide makes its way through the blood-brain barrier and into the body. This neuropeptide is now in the blood stream and influences the hormonal centers of the body. This is the biochemistry behind the science of psychoneuroimmunology.

Each of these hormonal centers are like tiny, individual brains in the body, and each carries a specific energy and frequency. Remember that frequency carries information. These hormonal centers of the body that neuropeptides influence are the thyroid gland in the throat, the thymus gland in the center of the chest, the adrenal gland just below the sternum in the pit of the gut, the digestive and pancreatic glands behind, and just below the naval and the sexual glands in the testes of a male and the ovaries of a female. (We will go into greater detail of the hormonal centers of the body in section three.) The hormones and chemicals released from these hormonal centers of our body are responsible for either creating a balance or imbalance of health within us. If they are on point, functioning at their highest potential, we are vibrant and healthy and the individual cells of the hormonal centers are manufacturing new and resilient proteins. If they are imbalanced, fatigued, and driven by stress, the individual hormonal centers are making fewer and weaker proteins.

Here is an example of how this mind-body experience works. You are out shopping for groceries and a drop-dead gorgeous man or woman walks right past you looking you directly in your eyes. This person is stunningly beautiful, so much so that you cannot get the image of them out of your mind. You suddenly start to have sexual thoughts involving the memory of this person. Your body gets warm and flushed, your heart races, you feel your reproductive centers turning on as blood starts to fill their tissues. You are having a full-on bodily experience based on the thought alone of this gorgeous person. The thought created a specific blend of chemicals released from the neuron synapses, which then influenced the limbic brain to create a specific blend of neuropeptides, which then flooded your bloodstream into the hormonal centers of your reproductive organs, turning your body on as if it were time to create a baby. Point to be made here is that your thoughts directly influence the cells in your body.

Stress happens in an almost limitless variety, but it can be broken down into three different categories. The first is physical stress, which happens to the body when there is a bodily injury like a broken bone from a fall or a torn ACL while playing a sport. The second is chemical stress, which comes from our environment causing a stress response in our body. Chemical stresses come from the toxins in air pollution, chemicals sprayed on our food and put in our food, cigarette smoke, etc. And the third form is emotional stress, like the loss of a loved one or a pet, a divorce, break up or getting fired from your job. From each of these forms of stress the body is receiving and then processing the autonomic reaction to the stress.

Humans are the only species to experience stress in such a psychological/emotional way. Most all other species only deal with an acute form of stress when some sort of threat to their survival causes them to react and escape. After the threat is avoided, the animal bounces right back into homeostasis. Whereas, we allow our co-worker in the cubical next to us to drive us into madness all day long. This in turn keeping our mind and body in the fight-or-flight state.

Over time, all these forms of stress turn into emotional stress as the body does not know the difference between the three categories. All the body knows is the hormonal and chemical response it is receiving cellularly as the brain responds to the stressor.

Think about a time when you were injured. Maybe you experienced some excruciating back pain? Or you broke your ankle? After the physical stress response to this injury, the body immediately starts to heal, but you cannot move the way you used to because of pain and doctor's orders. After three weeks of not being able to go for a run because of the pain or not be able to participate in your favorite activity because of the crutches, you start to feel down in the dumps. "This sucks! I cannot do what I want to do." You now feel angry and sad. The injury (physical stress is now an emotional stress). Your body is objective, so it does not know the difference between the two.

The same thing happens with chemical stress. For example, the corn that our favorite bag of chips is made from is being sprayed with a toxic chemical to keep the bugs from eating the corn. But for some reason we have a terrible headache and cannot focus like we want to. This headache is so random, and we cannot figure it out. Unbeknownst to us, the toxicity of the remnants of the chemical used on the corn is causing a stress response cellularly as these chemicals are signaling our cell that something's wrong. A specific inflammatory gene is programmed and released in large amounts into our bloodstream. This headache is so annoying, and we cannot focus to do our work during the day. Ugh! Anger and frustration lead to feelings of anxiety. "What if something is wrong with me?" "Why do I always have a headache?" "What if I have a brain tumor?" The chemical stressor of the chips has now been turned into an emotional stress of worry and fear.

If this is not bad enough, there is also a negative feedback loop that is a result of the stressor becoming chronic. For example, we will continue to use the model of the emotional stress from a fear of the headache hypothetically being made up by our mind as a possible brain tumor. This chemical signature of the fear and anxiety creates a biochemical imbalance in our body. This anxiety causes the hormones of cortisone and adrenaline to disrupt the balance of our body enough and create physical muscle tightness in our upper trapezius muscles and neck muscles.

The prolonged response to the stress causes tightness in our neck. Now, unconsciously, we are caught in a negative feedback loop. The emotional stress we are experiencing is creating physical stress in our neck and cervical spine as the fight or flight nervous system is not being turned off. Then we become worried about our neck pain as it is affecting our daily functions like driving our car and waking us up at night. We worry about how we will be able to function during the day with so much pain. And the negative feedback loop snowballs without our awareness of what is happening.

Caught in a loop of stress, it has become chronic. Everything in our life is stressful, hurrying to work, hurrying to get home, hurrying to cook dinner, hurrying to watch our favorite show and then hurrying to bed. Our bank account not having enough money in it, our daughter getting exposed to gossip at school, our co-worker driving us bonkers, our mother being diagnosed with cancer. Stress, stress and more stress. As the hormones of stress continually flood the cells of our body and with this continued flood of stress hormones, these cells become accustomed to the chemical signature. When we decide we want to change our lifestyle or habit that we know we need to change, our body gets a new chemical signature different from our habitual stressful thoughts, and then our body throws a fit.

It says, "Hey where is my anger?" or "Hey, where is my guilt?" "Hey, where is my worry?" because it has become addicted to this chemical signature of fear.

This is why habits are so hard to break. Below our conscious awareness, our body is sending signals via the spinal cord back up to the brain to say hey we need some more thoughts that we are used to. C'mon! This is what we know and is familiar to us. This is the ego, and the ego's job is to keep us in the known parts of everything. It throws an uprising in the form of excuses and uncomfortableness in the body when we sway from the known of our anxiety and worry. When confronted with change, either by our choice or not, chaos in our body ensues.

When we go into the unknown of a new way of eating, trying to meditate or change our state of being, the ego says, "oh, hell no!" and it makes us feel distressed. You may have heard the saying, learn to feel comfortable feeling uncomfortable. This is gold. Because if you can sit in the fire that the ego is going to have the body throw at you, but this time with an understanding of what is actually going on, you will see the beauty of what is on the other side.

At some point we have to sit in the fire of the great unknown and face our fears. If you are scared, it is ok. This is normal, just lean into it. Do not turn your cheek to it like we have been conditioned. We have done this entirely too much in our lives. Now is the time. There is never a better time than now. Trust that by the end of this book you will have the knowledge, comprehension and inspiration to take action and step into the fire of change.

The biochemistry of chronic stress is feeding our body a heavy dose of cortisol and adrenaline. As we learned before in the acute response of a life-threatening event, the release of these two hormones is essential. In the short term they upregulate essential functions of our body so we can run, hide or fight. But, when the stress hormones are being pumped out chronically every time we get angry at our co-worker for his opinion of the US government or the fear of money being low in our bank account, then we are on a fast track to pain and dis-ease. The overabundance of cortisol and adrenaline is chronically increasing our heart rate, while concomitantly increasing our blood pressure. This is what the body becomes accustomed to. This is what we know. And the ego wants to keep us there because it knows this familiar state of being.

As this happens most of our waking day, the increased blood pressure and heart rate causes our blood to crash into the bifurcation of our arterial walls at a very high pressure. A bifurcation is where the artery splits in two, sending blood into other artery pathways, similar to a fork in a river. Imagine a flood has occurred, and this river is flowing much faster. The water will be crashing into the bank of the river at the Y split and will cause the riverbank to break down, maybe even taking some trees and rocks with it down the stream.

This is a great analogy of what happens in our arteries. The constant increase of blood flow on these bifurcations causes the arteries to harden as their muscle wall must strengthen to withstand the increase flow and pressure. Consequently, plaque occurs on the artery wall as the body's response of trying to heal this constant pressure. As we continue to live by the hormones of stress, the plaque of the arterial wall cannot withstand the elevated pressure of blood crashing into it, and the plaque breaks away just like the riverbank rocks and trees. Now we have a major problem in our blood stream as these plaques can cause major damage, such as a heart attack or stroke. This is just one example of the many possibilities of stress causing dis-ease in our bodies.

In the next chapter, you will learn how to become conscious of all the thoughts and feelings running your program subconsciously. We will gain a better understanding of how to become aware of them and how they are a perfect spring board into your healthy, wealthy and pain-free dream life.

## Stress and its Effects on Proper Digestion

Most importantly, we need to realize that when we are living by the hormones of stress, our body couldn't care less about digesting the food we just ate. If we do not shine the light on how stress is running the show in our body, all the other solutions to healing and sealing our gut are merely passersby—even if we are eating the most perfect diet.

It makes sense that food would not be properly digested in stress because in order to increase our chances of survival from what our body perceives as a bear attack, we must utilize as much energy as possible to be transferred to our leg muscles, heart and brain. Therefore, all that energy we would normally use for proper food digestion is rerouted to our survival mechanisms.

When we understand that the surface area of the small intestines when unfolded and spread out would be the size of a tennis court, it is easy to see how much energy the digestive system requires to break down food. This is a massive surface of intestinal tissues all folded up inside our belly. There are literally trillions of cells working in our gut all for our greater good. Many of these cells are our own, but even more of them are other organisms living in our gut in a symbiotic relationship. We have named this tiny little eco-system of organisms the microbiome. Either way, whether they are our own cells or not, having proper energy distribution to them is essential for everything in the gut to function optimally. The digestive system is incredible, and the extent to how well it is functioning can be the difference between optimal health and dis-ease.

Throughout the majority of our day, it is our own habitual thinking triggering a chronic stress response. So now the amount of energy, which we need to splice and break down all the plentiful nutrients of the huge daily salad we ate for lunch is not sent to our gut. The energy is sent elsewhere. This leaves our digestion up to chance; who knows what goodness of vitamins, minerals and wholesome nutrition we are going to get from our conscious decision to eat a healthy lunch. If we are too busy worrying about the amount of money it cost us at Whole Foods, we are undoubtedly not getting the most out of our last meal. What happens when the cells in our digestive tract do not have the energy they need to function properly? Yep, you guessed it. Dis-ease occurs either in our gut itself or any other parts of the body.

You see, when we are stressed and our gut is not getting the vital life force energy it needs, our food does not break down properly and stays in bigger chains or clumps. We do not have the energy capacity to make all the enzymes needed to chop the food particles into pieces that come with a properly functioning digestive system. Even before we take a bite of food, we create the enzymes that help break down the food into smaller, more digestible pieces. But without the proper amount of energy distribution, our cells are not pumping out enough of the enzymes we need to properly break our food down. These big particles we just ate need to be unfolded and broken down into smaller pieces and chains of proteins, carbohydrates and fats. This allows both our own cells and the cells of the microbiome to recognize and utilize these broken-down parts. Without the proper breakdown, we have unrecognizable large clumps of food and toxins potentially entering into our bloodstream. This creates an immune response to attack and get rid of these unrecognizable foreign invaders, but when stress is running our body's program, the immune system takes a back seat as well.

In order to understand how improperly digested large clumps get into our bloodstream and how the immune system works directly with this process, we need to zoom in on the anatomy of the gut lining. At the cellular level, the intestinal wall is made up of tiny cells called enterocytes. Enterocytes fit together side-by-side like vertical bricks making a wall throughout the entire intestinal tract. These brick-like cells are held together by their cell membranes similar to the way Velcro sticks together. This Velcro-like connection of the enterocytes is called the tight junctions. On the heads of blocks of the enterocytes are tiny fingers of cilia called the microvilli. This creates a brush border helping to move the digestion process along down the intestinal track. Take a look at figure 3 to see an image of the enterocyte. These cells line the entire inside of the intestinal tube, and food moves slowly through this tube in the same way a slight clog travels through a pipe.

The astonishing thing is the enterocyte lining is only one cell thick. On the underside of the one-celled-thick lining is our bloodstream. This means the barrier between our bloodstream (the inside of our body) and our intestinal tract (the outside world) is one cell thick. The thickness of one cell keeps the outside world from seeping into our inside world.

Throughout the entire intestinal wall, there are wavelike protrusions of tissues made up of these enterocytes going up and down like a roller coaster. The wall consists of millions of folds on top of folds, creating wave-like tissue flowing down into low valleys and then up and into a peak again. This gives the intestinal lining a greater surface area without taking up so much space. This phenomenon reminds me of the fractal patterns we see in nature. Like the waves in a ripple of water or the spiraling of a snail shell. You will see these folds in figure 4.

In each of these crevasses and on top of the fingers (cilia) of the intestinal wall are the home to trillions and trillions of tiny bacteria of the microbiome. Micro meaning microscopic and biome meaning living organism. These tiny living organisms are composed of bacteria, fungi, protozoa, yeasts, etc. all living inside our very own gut.

All these teeny things are simply using our intestinal tract as a host. In the waves of folds and throughout the cilia of the enterocytes, the trillions of bacteria of the microbiome live in a layered coating of mucus. The mucous coats the top of the enterocyte cell wall lining throughout all the millions of folds of intestinal tissue. Cells within the interaction lining called goblet cells secrete this mucus that the microbiome live in and to help food pass down throughout the intestinal tract. With a healthy, diverse bacterial population, this mucosal lining creates an extended protective barrier all around the cylindrical digestive tract.

When these tiny bacteria are in a good balance having a proper ratio of a diverse number of species, they work for the greater good of our body. The microbiome and its ecosystem within us and on us is directly connected to our health. However, because of its sheer magnitude in the number of organisms, it dwarfs our own human cells in comparison. Consequently, because they are so small and exist in such magnitude, we are only now beginning to gather the data needed to better understand this ancient life living in us. Yet we have learned that we absolutely rely on them for our moment-to-moment health, and we do not ever need to fear them and demonize them. For without them, we simply would not be living as the human species. However, because of the overuse of antibiotics in food, medicine and soaps, their diversity is being violated in much of our population. We will take a closer look at the brilliant communication network between the microbiome

and our brain in Section three with the discussion of our second
energy center.

# Enterocyte

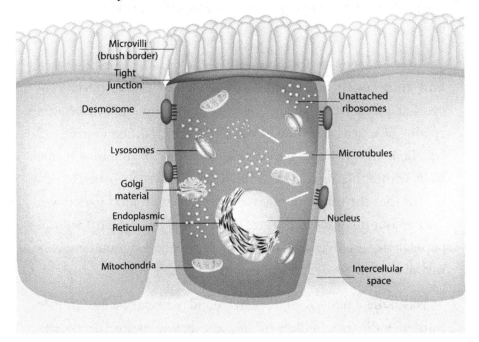

*Figure 3*

During the digestive process, the bacteria feed off the nutrients
in the food making its way down the tract. As they eat, digest and
then excrete food we ate, they make all sorts of very important
life-sustaining vitamins, minerals and chemicals for our body to
utilize for health. These nutrients gradually make their way down
through layers of the mucous lining where more bacteria feed and
excrete their wastes in a totem pole like fashion. The end product
(i.e., the bacteria's poop) then either gets absorbed into our enterocyte cells or passed on down the intestinal tube. The enterocytes
take important nutrients into the cell to make more life-sustaining
proteins for exportation into the blood stream.

# SMALL INTESTINE

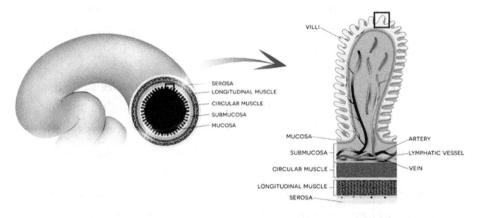

**SMALL INTESTINE**

**A FOLD OF THE INTESTINAL LINING**

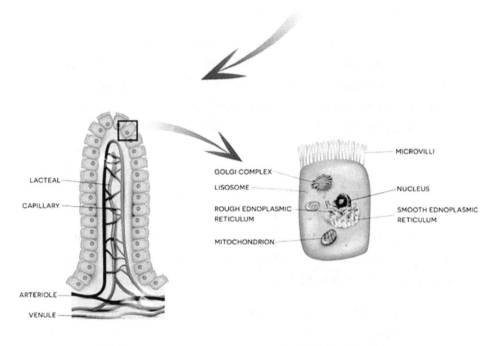

**VILLI**

**EPITHELIAL CELL**

*Figure 4*

As you can gather, a balanced and diverse ecosystem within our gut is extremely important to overall health. On the other hand, when we are living in chronic stress and the body is mobilizing all its life-sustaining energy *away* from our internal organs, rerouting it for our survival, the digestion of the last meal we ate, that is now in our intestines, gets put on the back burner.

Day in and day out as we live in this hurry-up, stressful state, the tissues of our gut simply do not get what they need. Our microbiome takes a huge hit because of the sympathetic nervous system rerouting the energy it requires to function optimally. Additionally, we now have large molecules of food unrecognized by the body. Not only is there too little energy available for the tissues of the intestines to function as needed, there is also not enough energy for the immune system that lives in and around all the tissues of the gut to properly deal with the harmful agents.

Eighty percent of our immune system is found around our intestines to protect us from the chemicals, toxins, carcinogens, etc., that are coming into our intestines from the outside world. Without adequate energy for this defense, the intestinal tissues become inflamed and start to break down. The mucous lining of the microbiome begins to dry up, losing its balanced ecosystem of diverse bacteria, allowing opportunistic fungi, like candida albicans to overgrow. Now without this proper coating of mucus, another line of defense in the gut is diminished, and this allows these large undigested particles, toxins and many other inflammation sparking molecules like lipopolysaccharides to easily access the blood stream, bumping right up to the enterocyte-lined tissue.

As this breakdown ensues, the Velcro like connection of the tight junctions starts to peel apart thanks to the inflammation caused by the combination of stress, toxins in our food, depleted mucus and imbalance of microbiome. The immune system cannot keep up with the needs of repair and regeneration, and the tissues of the gut lining start to leak. This is what is known as leaky gut. We simply do not have the energy, nutrients or proper digestion in our gut to take care of business. Now there is space between the enterocytes allowing for toxins to seep straight into the bloodstream and lymph system.

Have a look in figure 4 at how the veins and the arteries are directly underneath the epithelial cells. In healthy intestinal tissue the enterocytes deliver whatever the body needs through the cell itself into the bloodstream. However, with a leaky gut, the outside world is able to enter directly into our bloodstream. Now toxins, large food particles, non-beneficial bacteria, fungi and viruses are all able to sneak into our system. Not only does this cause inflammation and dis-ease in the intestinal tissue itself, but it literally opens the floodgates for potential dis-ease anywhere in the body. With these toxins in our blood stream, they go wherever the blood goes. Now, these inflammatory agents having free access to the inner world of our body causes a dis-ease cascade throughout the body.

Think of all the chronic dis-eases prevalent today. From the autism spectrum to allergies. From irritable bowel syndrome to heart dis-ease. The inflammation coming in from our toxic environment and leaking through our gut is causing the chronic dis-ease epidemic in our population today. Remember, 60% of our population has to deal with a chronic dis-ease. Think of the resolution to these problems if we simply stopped the leakage of our gut.

As you can see, living in chronic stress is bad enough for our gut health and furthermore our overall health, but now let us throw in the food most Americans are eating in the Standard American Diet. As you will become very familiar with in great detail in section four, what most Americans are eating does not even deserve the title of food. I call it "not food." This is because the body hardly recognizes the hyper-caloric, over processed and nutrient depleted Franken food so easily accessible in today's world. It works out perfectly that the acronym for the Standard American Diet happens to be SAD.

We now have a tired, inflamed, run-down gut, working at 20% of its maximum capacity (thanks to stress) combined with a depleted mucous lining of the gut that can hardly protect our delicate enterocytes from the extremely toxic food coming from our SAD. This is obviously a lose-lose scenario. Keep reading because it does not stop here.

Because the "not food" of the SAD is so high in sugar, processed corn and processed wheat (all broken down into high amounts of sugar), the non-beneficial bacteria and fungi (like candida albicans) start to overgrow and take over the territory of our gut. These opportunistic organisms thrive off sugar. And with little counterbalance of their opposing beneficial bacteria, fungi, etc., the dis-ease causing, non-beneficial organisms rule the territory of the intestines.

When they are overgrown, they become very hungry and vocal to our brain. They crave the simple sugars, and they send text messages to the brain via the Vagus nerve to tell our brain to give them more carbohydrates (sugars). Just think about how powerful food cravings are. I do not know about you, but I have driven miles just to have that pizza I was craving. We get hit with this food craving all without our conscious awareness, and we act fast because this craving is loud in our brain.

Moreover, the crops processed to make the food of the SAD are heavily sprayed with a toxin called glyphosate. This is the active chemical found in Roundup®. This chemical is actually an antibiotic, which in turn kills even more of the beneficial bacteria in our gut along with a bucket list of other dis-ease causing side effects. So now with the little energy our gut has to repair and regenerate, in combination with the antibiotic-laced food of the SAD, the tissues of our gut and its microbiome partners are between the hammer and the anvil.

On top of all this, chronic stress causes the release of glucocorticoids into our system. Glucocorticoids are a classification of hormones like adrenaline and cortisol. These glucocorticoids contain an appetite-stimulating component to them in order to replace all the energy of the perceived threat of the lion attacking us. There is no lion—just our mind having bursts of intermittent stressful thoughts of our co-worker's terrible choice of outfit today. The glucocorticoids released into the bloodstream take time to return to normal, which means that while they hang around, they are stimulating our appetite.

When our appetite increases, we generally crave carbohydrates: breads, sugar, crackers, chips and candy. And again, thanks to the SAD, these foods are right at our fingertips. Now the abundance of these carbohydrates (simple sugars) causes a flood of glucose in the blood stream. With such an excess amount of calories in the blood, the body must store this overload somewhere. It is stored in our body fat. As this chronic stress cycle continues, we continue to eat the easy and readily accessible "not food" that is in our face from TV, billboards, social media ads, etc. every day, and our cells become flooded with glucose.

Now the hormone Insulin is secreted in response to elevated glucose levels in our bloodstream. One of insulin's main jobs is to tell the cell to take in glucose. Insulin is like a key that opens a locked door, allowing glucose to come into the cell. Glucose is like gasoline to an engine, inside the cell it goes through a combustion process, giving our bodies energy. When we are eating this hypercaloric, high sugar (glucose) "not food" for every meal plus snacks between meals, our cells start to resist the flood of glucose coming in. The cell has enough, and it does not allow insulin to open the door and allow glucose in. This is the beginnings of insulin resistance, pre-diabetes and type 2 diabetes. Now glucose is in elevation in the bloodstream, and this causes even more dis-ease.

In section four we will dive into the dis-ease causing effects of glycation, which is the result of the elevated insulin and glucose in the blood.

Now we have a number of psychological triggers sending our brain messages below our conscious awareness. These unconscious triggers are in no particular order.

1. Glucocorticoids in the blood causing hunger while messaging our brain to refuel with starches.

2. Eating dopamine producing foods (foods that are high in carbohydrate) to fill an emotional void from the chronic stress.

3. A sugar crash from the last high-carbohydrate meal, triggering our brain that we are hungry again as the cells and the candida albicans send messages to the brain to "FEED ME."

We gorge ourselves in order to offset the feelings of our terrible day. Just to get that temporary satisfaction of dopamine in the brain desperately trying to fill the void, all the while being unaware of this program running in our subconscious. This is known as emotional eating, and living in chronic stress is the culprit.

My hope is that you can see the writing on the wall. Stress causes the vital energy needed for proper digestion to be mismanaged for what the body perceives as its more important survival function. When the limited blood and therefore energy are not sent to the digestive system, the cells of the digestive track are not at their peak performance. When cells are not at their peak performance and working collectively as a team, they get selfish and function more as individuals than as a unit. Without the proper energy to work optimally, the cells left in survival mode become selfish as they cannot rely on the system, so they are forced to only care for themselves. Chaos and entropy soon follow suit. Energetically these cells are incoherent and out of rhythm. Then throw in the SAD, laced with glyphosate and combined with enough sugar in one meal for an entire week's worth of meals, we are straight lining it to dis-ease.

Here's a flowchart in no particular order, except that stress kicks it all off, to help you see the trickle-down effect of just a fraction of what the gut is going through.

Stress reroutes energy from the gut

Not enough energy in the gut to digest food properly

Leaving large particles of food undigested

Body not absorbing important nutrients already

Without adequate energy tissues begin
to break down, causing inflammation

Eat toxic SAD causing insults
to already inflamed tissue

Microbiome loses diversity as mucus depletes,
in turn exposing delicate enterocyte cell wall

Leaks in the epithelial lining occur

Toxins, undigested food, unwanted bacteria,
etc. seep into the bloodstream

Creating more inflammation and
starting systemic inflammation

Immune system cannot keep up

SAD is loaded with sugar,
causing blood sugar spikes

Glycation and more inflammation
in brain and body as a result of high glucose

Chronic stress flooding body with
glucocorticoids cause carbohydrate
rich food cravings

SAD fills this emotional and chemical void

Being unaware, the cycle continues to worsen

## Stress Out—Love of Life In

The procedures outlined in this section are based on the work of Joe Dispenza.[6]

In this section, I will teach you why it is so hard to change. You will learn why so many times your attempts at changing some aspect of your life have fallen short. First, we will learn in order to change we must alter our energy and therefore our state of being by making a firm decision. I will take you through the steps of determining the status quo of what state of being is running your existing body and mind program. In this step, you will gain awareness to recognize what the problem is. As you become more and more familiar with the states of being that have been running your unconscious program, I will then lead you through the steps of integrating and releasing these unwanted programs that have become your normal state of being.

After you have determined the status quo, you will then determine the target of what and who you want to be. The new you. You will create the absolute greatest version of yourself. In this process you will practice the integration of how to recalibrate your body to a new way of being. You will get clear on what you want in your life and how the new you will think, act and feel. After working through the clutter of the old self and determining what your new self will be, we will learn the role that epigenetics and psychoneuroimmunology play in your new state of health. You will understand how if chronic stress can create pain and disease, then the coherent and rhythmic heartfelt emotions of love and worthiness being the new status quo will do the opposite and create health, wellness and abundance in your life. And finally, I will teach you how to meditate. I will show you that you *can* meditate (despite what you may believe) and that many of us have a misrepresentation of what it means to meditate. I will provide you with alternate types of meditation to help you find the one that is the best fit for yourself.

## Why is change so hard?

How many times have you tried to change a habit in your life you know you should not be doing only to find yourself a few days, weeks or months later going right back to that bad habit?

To change is very difficult. There is no other way around it. And to create a change in our life it takes a massive amount of energy.

Now that you know how the hormones of stress create an addiction in the cells of your body, you can start to piece together why changing something you know you should not be doing is so hard. Our body becomes accustomed to the chemical signature being sent to it on a daily basis. This addiction becomes our unconscious program that runs us.

Using sugary treats after dinner as an example, we know we should not eat the ice cream or the mini-Snickers bars every night for dessert because it is not beneficial to our health. But, as much as we know this philosophically, we still cannot stop eating it. Why is this? We now understand how stress and intestinal incoherence play into the strong carbohydrate cravings, but let us take a closer look at the emotional component of this addiction.

We have to understand that everything we do in a form of a habit is for an emotional pay-off. We choose the ice cream because it makes us feel a certain way. Maybe we get relief when we feel the satisfaction of the dopamine and serotonin being released in our brain when the body receives its fix of the ice cream. Or maybe we feel joy and comfort that fills a void within us from the ice cream. Whatever the feeling is does not necessarily matter. The point is that this outside source is what we are using to create a certain feeling inside our body.

In the upcoming written work, we are going to go through step-by-step, we will first unpack some of these behaviors we are choosing to take part in that we no longer want to. We will shine light on the subconscious thoughts, feeling and behaviors that drive these unwanted habits. Furthermore, we will learn that with our own free will, we can create these satisfying feelings of love, happiness, gratitude and joy with no external source needed. All we need is a clear vision of the possibility of a future that inspires us to feel these elevated emotions.

We must realize that subconsciously, we are searching for something outside our body to create a feeling inside our body. Through psychoneuroimmunology this creates a message to our cells. And epigenetically, this then signals the cell on what protein to create or not create. This is where having the knowledge of what is happening meets the awareness of catching ourselves in the subconscious act. We can only catch this happening by raising awareness of our current behaviors.

Inside our little box of consciousness that we are stuck in and cannot see out of, is the belief that the ice cream is bringing us joy and relief. Most of the time, after the emotional payoff runs out, we feel guilt and shame for being overcome by the addiction. The psychoneuroimmunologic chemical signature of guilt and shame further the epigenetic signals to the cell that are deleterious to our health. As well as sucking us back into another old subconscious program of feeling guilt and shame toward our behaviors.

When we have made up our mind to change, we have become aware that nothing new has happened in our life, and we are tired of it. When nothing new is happening in our life, this is because the way we think and the way we feel have not changed. We are stuck in the status quo of our habitual behaviors. If nothing is changing, then we are feeling the same emotions in our life every day. Our emotions are created from past events in our lives. The stronger the amplitude of energy from the past event, the stronger the emotion. When we are living the same life every day, our body is getting the same chemical signature day in and day out. Epigenetically, the same genes are being created, which creates wear and tear, resulting in weaker proteins to go to work in our body. Our body becomes addicted to the past, and it does not want to change because the past is familiar. You know, when it feels good to be angry sometimes? That is an old behavior our ego does not want to change because it knows it and is addicted to it.

The brain's primary job is to remember; it recalls all the things we have learned to date. The stronger the emotion, the more we will remember the event. It is important to understand that this is true for both positive and negative events. This is a great thing when it comes to our survival. We can recall a memory with a strong emotion attached to all the things that could potentially be fatal to our survival. Like the time we were searching for shelter in the cave, and we found a bear living inside. That scared us so badly we will never enter that cave again. Subconsciously, we know that, and the emotion of fear created in our body when we saw that bear is branded into our brain very deeply. We will never go there again! Ancestrally, this was great for our survival. It kept us alive.

But today, now that we are living in a world that is safe and sound, living in houses where we do not have to worry about a bear, our deeply branded survival emotions are created in a totally different way. Today, fear is created by things like the failure of not making enough money to pay for our mortgage, comparing ourselves to being not as cool as the famous people on Instagram, and getting made fun of at school.

So, if we want to make a change in our life like quitting our sugar addiction, we must have knowledge of how to do so. Our body becomes addicted to this feeling the ice cream creates. This is the thinking and feeling, feeling and thinking feedback loop. When the body does not have its chemical signature the ice cream gives it, the body starts to send messages to the brain. Now the body has become the instigator by sending signals to the brain through the Vagus nerve, saying, "hey where's my hit of the chemicals that the ice cream creates?" The brain gives in and starts thinking of what it knows creates those feelings. ICE CREAM! And without being aware of this, you find yourself right back in the habit of eating ice cream, only later going to bed feeling awful about yourself because you gave in to the temptation. Telling yourself, "I'll just change tomorrow."

On a side note, our body has been made to reward us for sugary, high-calorific foods in order to ensure our survival. Our evolution has been dependent on our ancestors making the best choice of high-calorie, high-nutrient foods to make it through the times of famine. For example, when our ancestors found a beehive honeycomb, they gorged themselves on it as a treat because honey did not come around very often. We were made to be rewarded for foods like this by our brain sending us dopamine signals to remember this food, where it came from, what it tastes like and that it made us ecstatic.

But the problem in today's world is that food companies know how this reward system works, and they make "not food" in a lab that is chemically processed to have the perfect ratios of sugar, protein and fat, making it nearly impossible for us to say no. The packaging, television advertising and shelf placement at the grocery store are all specially designed to trigger the subconscious reward centers in our brain, making such food highly addictive. Keep in mind that we will talk about this in more detail in Section Four.

81

## The Ego and Change

The ego has a big problem with change. To change is to enter the unknown. We have not done it yet, so the ego does not know what to expect. This rattles the ego's cage. It stirs it up, and the ego does not like to be bothered. It likes to be lazy because being lazy is the known. The ego loves to control. It loves to be able to predict. And to control is to be able to predict the future. There is no better way to anticipate the future than by living in the same way you have in your past. This is safe for the ego, so it makes it very hard for you to venture away from your habits. Ever wonder why we are all such control freaks? Well, now you know.

The minute you say you want to change, the ego gets rattled, and it is going to throw everything it has at you in the form of excuses not to do it. It is going to make the past (the known) feel so good and comfortable. Whereas, the unknown will seem very scary and dark. The ego will sway you back to safety. The ego will say, "no way—do not change, that does not feel right." In the unknown because of the ego's tricks, you will feel a sense of chaos and uneasiness as you think about change. This is how the ego wins and gets you to go back to living your past all over again. Staying stuck in the same old status quo, just wishing and hoping.

What we need to be aware of is the fact that we are not going to die if we change. The ego makes us believe that—so we decide not to change. But when we take that first step into the unknown, we now have taken our power back. And we now are in control of our future. Remember the observer effect and how powerful our focused attention is? It can change nothing into something. However, I should not call this nothing because it is actually not nothing. It is actually a field of inexhaustible energy that is always there. We only call it nothing because we cannot see it with our eyes or touch it with our hands or hear it or… You get the point. In the unknown, when we place our attention on what we choose with our own free will, like our dream life that we desire, we are creating it with our own inherent power of focused attention. This instantly switches us to become the creators of our life as opposed to being the victims of it. We have that choice. And we are the only one that does. No one, no thing or no place can do this for us.

Just on the other side of the ego's attempt to make us think we will die if we try to change is freedom, peace, joy and bliss. But we must take that first step into fear and show the ego it is not in charge. We are.

In order to make this change we have so desperately tried to create we have to get serious and make up our minds that we are going to change. This decision must rock our body so hard it creates a memorable amount of energy to catapult the change process. We have to be extremely inspired to change.

## Making Up Your Mind

First, you must make a definite decision. You must know specifically what you want to change. What is it in your life that you are not happy with and want to change? This decision must have serious energy behind it. This decision must carry enough energy to alter your body chemically. Most of the time, we wait for crisis in our life to create enough chaos that we have no choice but to take a closer look at ourselves from an observer's perspective. In the failed attempts to change previously in our life, we have talked ourselves out of it. Our ego kicks in and says, "Oh just wait 'til tomorrow." Or "Who do you think you are to be able to do that? You cannot do that." We now know the ego does not like change. When we are living in our mind and driven by our ego, we try to predict every outcome in our life. We have been conditioned to everything known (our habits). We now have the power of awareness to understand what is happening that keeps us from changing.

Therefore, get clear and specific on what you want to change. What do you want in your life that you do not have? What change do you want to see in the world? What is the first step to make this change? When you are clear, you can start to work toward creating the change. This change has to charge us up. We have to get big, think big and be greater than the old self that wants to sit on the couch and eat potato chips. We must create energy. By using our frontal lobe, and becoming aware that we have free will, we can do anything when we change our energy.

Just think about something in your life that you have already created. You made up your mind. You made a hard-set decision that you were going to do this. No maybe, no procrastination, just pure motivation and desire. This is the fuel that ignites the change. You don't have to wait on some external circumstance to make a change. You simply just make a firm decision. We do this naturally, we are creators. Just look at all the current technology around you. We humans were the responsible conduit for the creation of this.

When we make up our mind with such great energy, then we are no longer going to be a victim to our environment, body or time. This decision sends a chemical signature to our cells that switches on the energy we need to carry out the change. In other words, the firm decision is creating a chemical change in our body through psychoneuroimmunology. It is flipping the switch to catapult us into greatness, and we are now signaling our genes in a different way through epigenetics. We have changed the environment within our body.

## Determining Status Quo

Now that you have made up your mind, you must know what the problem is in order to fix it. What are the bad habits we know we need to change? What are our habits and behaviors we are not proud of? What are the things we feel guilty for doing or not doing? Is there anger and rage in our life we cannot seem to suppress? Do we have judgement and hate we cannot believe we still harbor? We are now going to take a hard look at who we've been.

You learned in Section One how much we are living in the chemical signature of stress. It should make sense, then, if you want to live a pain free and healthy life, you must be aware of what and who you do NOT want to be. If 95% of our mind is a subconscious program, then to transform, we have to become aware of who we are that 95% of the time. By recognizing this, we are becoming conscious of our subconscious programs.

These upcoming questions are very tough to reflect on, but if we want to change, we have to realize how we have been thinking, acting and feeling. For most of us, the stress hormones run our lives for the greater part of the day. We must shine light on them in order to know they exist. Otherwise, they are hidden and running in the background, sending the stress chemicals throughout our body without us ever being aware of them.

We need to know what emotions this habit we want to change creates. We need to take a really close look at our life and ask ourselves some questions like these coming up. Reflecting on what we are doing on a moment-to-moment basis, we become aware of who we are when the status quo is running on autopilot. We use the frontal lobes of our brain and think about who we are being when this unwanted, unconscious program is running behind our awareness. We must face the challenge of doing the elusive self-reflection.

What does it mean to reflect on ourselves? We must begin to look at our life as if we were someone else observing ourselves. What kind of person do they see? What are the behaviors of this person? How do they act? The human brain is amazing, and it has the ability for us to look at ourselves from the outside in. Through what is called metacognition, we humans have a super power of being aware that we are aware. We can learn to use this super-power to our advantage and become super aware of our default mode actions and behaviors.

To do this, we must go within and listen to what arises. This takes a great will and a lot of courage. Our ego comes back into our mind and tries again to knock us off track of finding out who our true self really is. The ego does not want us to go down this road of self-reflection because it knows we will unseat it and want to change. So, the ego is going to make you think you are too weak to look within and reflect. It will do everything it can to keep you from finding out who you truly are. The ego will try to make you feel guilty for how you have been in your past. Saying things such as, "Oh, you have been such a terrible person." "How can you be so mean?" "Why would you want to reflect on all your negative traits?" Remember these familiar traits are what the ego knows, because these are the programs chemically influencing the cells of our body most of our day. The ego wants to keep you in these old emotions as it knows change is coming.

Not only this, but the ego plays tricks on us by using avoidance. For example, because you have now decided to make a change in your life, you will be going into the unknown, and we now know that the ego does not want anything to do with the unknown. In order to influence you away from change and the unknown, it will try its hardest to convince you to go make a drink, clean the house or some known, familiar thing that it already knows is safe. Anything to sway you away from doing the hard work of self-reflection. Being aware of this is your empowerment to work through it.

Self-reflection is a skill that, like any other skill, can be developed. It takes practice. As you practice and become better at this, you will see that you will be able to separate your conscious mind from your subconscious mind. The autopilot behaviors and habits will start to come into your awareness, and you will catch them before they happen. This is where you start to take your innate power back. You now have a choice to be these old habitual behaviors or not.

The best way to find out who we have been and what it is exactly about ourselves that we want to change is to ask ourselves some questions that make our frontal lobes become more aware.

We are so caught up in the program of our society, family, job, etc. that we rarely take time to use our frontal lobe and ask big questions that deep down we're all connected to. Things like, who am I? What is my purpose on this planet? Where did humans come from? What is the meaning of life? These questions are innate in all of us as we have forgotten who we truly are.

Take time to ask yourself these questions or questions like these and write all of this down on a sheet of paper or in a notebook.

Who am I?

How do I present myself to the world?

Am I being/acting how I want to be?

How would others explain who I am?

What masks do I wear so people cannot see the real me?

What is something about myself I would like to change?

Is there a difference between the person I present to others and the person I really am?

What feeling do I experience and struggle with throughout each day?

What do I hide from others?

If there is one thing I can change about myself, what would it be?

Now that you have taken a good look at your old self and recognize what kind of habits, beliefs and behaviors are running your state of being most of the time, it is time to look at the emotions connected with these familiar states. Read through these limited emotions below and pick one or two that resonate with you—meaning they have a charge in your body. You may find some that are not listed. No problem. Either way, write the emotion down as you will work with this emotion in further steps in this exercise. It is not so important to be specific with the exact emotion as it is to simply become aware of what program has been running. The whole point is to create awareness for yourself.

Insecurity, hatred, judgement, victimization, worry, guilt, depression, shame, anxiety, regret, suffering, frustration, fear, greed, sadness, disgust, envy, anger, resentment, unworthiness, jealousy, lack.

It is important to know all these emotions are linked to the stress hormones and chemically are influencing your body all the time. So, even though you might resonate with more than one emotion, try to stick with one as they all lead to a similar destructive stress hormone cocktail. As you continue with this work, you will find that new emotions may rise to the surface that you want to change, but you did not even realize were in your subconscious. In linear time, you will integrate those emotions through the meditation process.

For example, when I started this work, the emotion I became aware I was living with the most was insecurity. As I meditated on this emotion day after day, other emotions such as anxiety, jealousy, fear and anger all rose to my awareness of who I was being. I realized my insecurity is tied to my anxiety because when I am insecure of my true self and I am not rooted in my soul, then I am running on a program of what others think of me and wanting to gain their approval. This then causes anxiety in me as I go down the rabbit hole of "do they like me or do they think I'm stupid?" Likewise, I realized that my insecurity caused me to pick out my perceived faults in others to divert reflection of myself onto them. I would judge and hate others, thereby giving me an emotional payoff and worthiness because I'm perceiving the other person as inferior. As I have become more aware, I realize this is all linked to insecurity of my own true self. Furthermore, as I have integrated these insecurities, I can now catch myself habitually wanting to take part in the old programs and stop them in their tracks.

You will find that as you continue the work on the main emotion you picked, all the other emotions you may have resonated with or that arise in your awakening will all continue to lessen. Eventually you will see those emotions and catch them, but because of the practice and awareness you will feel no bond to them. You will simply observe them with no emotion connected to them. This is the purpose of this work. You are no longer controlled by the unconscious low emotion. Most importantly, you realize the only person you are affecting by living in that old emotional state is yourself.

Now that you have an emotion picked, it's time to sense how this unwanted emotion feels in your body. Do you feel it in your chest? Perhaps you feel the emotion up in your throat. Or the pit of your gut? Become aware of what part of your body this feeling manifests in. In this exercise, you must really focus and go within to feel where it is in your body that you have the feeling this emotion creates. Be with it, acknowledge it, and try not to judge it. Be the observer of it. Do this more and let everything that happens as you feel it in your body be ok.

This is challenging because the old you has done everything in its power NOT to feel this emotion by avoiding it. This feeling has nothing to do with your future, but this is who you have been, and it is running behind your awareness. This is the program you will reprogram. The attachment to this feeling keeps you stuck. This feeling has been created from an emotional reaction to a past event in your life, and the feeling has stuck and is now running your program. Remember that your body is receiving the chemical signature of this feeling, and the body has become addicted to these chemicals. This makes it extremely hard to change because the body is now conditioned to this old feeling that you really do not want to be feeling. But it has felt good to feel this way because the body gets its fix from feeling this way. The body has been influencing the mind to think and feel this way so it stays the same. Remember the tricks of the ego.

Now that you have the emotion and the feeling written down and reflected on where in your body it presents itself, you have important pieces of change identified. The next step is to describe what your state of being is when this emotion and feeling is running your system's program.

Ask yourself, "What thoughts am I thinking when I feel this way?" Ask yourself "What kind of attitude do I have when I am feeling insecure (or whatever emotion you chose)?"

As you ask yourself these questions, become aware of and remember your thoughts when you have this common emotion you want to change. What is your state of mind when this old program is on autopilot? This is your feeling and thinking, thinking and feeling feedback loop. Focus in with laser sharp concentration and really remember this state that runs your unconscious program.

Now write it down. Here are some examples of limited states of mind from which you can get a good idea of how you behave.

Competitive, overwhelmed, complaining, blaming, confused, distracted, self-pitying, desperate, lacking, overly intellectual, self-important, shy, timid, introverted, needing recognition, under or overconfident, lazy, dishonest, controlling, deceptive, conceited, dramatic, rushing, needy, self-involved, sensitive or insensitive.

Now it is time to admit who you have been and declare it verbally. By facing this truth of who you have been and admitting it, you are accepting vulnerability. Being vulnerable is taking off the masks you have been using to hide who you really are from the outside world. Admitting this emotion that has been running behind your awareness is not weakness. In fact, it is the ultimate strength. It is like standing up to a bully. This unwanted emotion has pushed you around and caused you to manipulate and control your life in a number of different ways. All so you did not have to face this unwanted emotion. It is time to take a stand. Admitting is true greatness.

In order to do this without feeling guilty, we must realize we are connecting and admitting to a higher universal consciousness. This is who I call God. There are many names for this same unconditional loving intelligence. A name can never do this universal mind that all life comes from any justice as this power is beyond our comprehension. It is possible to admit our failures and our faults as we realize this loving intelligence will never punish us, never judge us, never manipulate us, never abandon us, never blame us, never keep score on our mishaps, never reject us, never stop loving us and will never be separate from us. This is like falling into the softest, safest, pillow-like cloud you could ever imagine. It is the loving embrace from a mother and father of their newborn child at all times that never ends. It is the ultimate comfort, relief, safety and security.

We have been conditioned to believe we are not worthy, and we inherently have something wrong with us. We have been conditioned to believe it is bad to make mistakes, that only A's are good and C's, D's, and F's are a failure. We have been conditioned by a society that laughs at us when we fall, and this keeps us from trying to leap as we are afraid of being ridiculed. The loving universal intelligence behind all life that I call God would never laugh, judge or wrong us for this. This intelligence is loving us the whole way through, knowing that whatever happens to us is absolute perfection because it already knows everything about us. If it judged us, it would be judging itself because we are it and it is us.

Plain and simple, we are afraid to be wrong. We have grown up being shamed when we were wrong. Whether it was our parents yelling at us when we accidentally spilled something or our pastor telling us we would go to hell if we did something the Bible classified as a sin. This has put the fear of God in us. But in reality, there is no fear in God. Just love. This social conditioning has made it very hard to admit our mistakes. Many times, in the moment of doing something we are not proud of, we lie our way out of it rather than admitting what we have done. All to avoid the ridicule of the perceived wrong. This is avoidance. When we avoid who we truly have been for too long, this causes imbalance in our body and brain.

But when we muster up the courage to admit who we have been and what we have done that we feel guilty for, we start to free up some deeply rooted stuck energy. On the other side of the fear of admittance is freedom. The energy this emotion has used in our body is exhausting, and when we let this emotion go by admitting and declaring, we now have access to that available energy it has been using. This is something in my personal meditation sessions I absolutely love as I can physically feel the release of energy and a simultaneous gain of energy as I let it go.

Write it down.

Examples to admit to your higher power:

I have felt guilty for most of my life because I do not believe I am good enough.

I have lied to people about myself to make them think better of me.

I have felt sorry for myself for most of my life because I am blaming someone or something else.

I have felt like a failure, so I try extra hard to make the world believe I am smart, wealthy and successful.

I pretend to be happy so people do not know how I really feel inside.

Deep down, I am afraid to fall in love because I do not want to be hurt.

Time to announce out loud who you have been. In this part of the exercise, you actually verbalize the emotion you have been and that you want to change. Put it out there with your voice. Release this stuck energy from your body. Admit to this loving intelligence who you have been, for it can handle anything, and it will take this burden from you and integrate it seamlessly into the greater good of the universe. Let it go and say out loud whatever you have been afraid to say. This liberates so much energy because you are releasing this old emotional energy with your voice.

After you have said this out loud, you now can surrender. Feel that you are safe to let go of everything you think you need to be. Think of all the conditioning in your life that led you to this point. Let go of it. Think about how hard you have tried your whole life—trying so hard to be whatever you believed you needed to be. This is not good or bad, right or wrong. You have simply done your best. However, these burdens we have avoided are very heavy and energy consuming, so feel the relief that letting go of this heavy burden gives you. Just let it all go and melt into your chair. Surrender to the infinite intelligence, and trust that it knows exactly what to do with loving kindness.

As you surrender deeply, you are surrendering to love. In this loving intelligence there is no guilt, resentment, shame or any negative emotions you have been conditioned to feel when you admit or surrender something. There is no getting in trouble or consequences. The only result of this surrender is a deep relief in the act of letting go. The intelligence behind all of life loves you and that is it. It has no judgment toward you whatsoever. It accepts you for who you are on all levels. Deeply embodying this allows you to trust in a higher power. This is Divine order of all that is. Surrender to this love.

After you have admitted what you have done and own up to it, it is much easier to let go. When we put on masks and fake emotions in our lives only to please others, we are separating from our true self. We create a lot of resistance in the body because deep down in our truth, we know we are putting on a front in order to fit in. As we let go of this, we are letting go of control. We are accepting who we truly are. We remember to trust in something greater than the facade of the material world. This connects us to the truth of the universe. We feel safe. We can start to sense a feeling of being loved. We become worthy. We are enough. Energy comes back into our body and creates an amazing feeling of relief and safety.

This practice has helped me catch myself during my day when I fall into victim mode. Victim mode is when I allow something in my outer environment to determine my mood in my internal environment. I like to go to the bathroom or a private area to close my eyes and stop these old patterns with my free will as much as I can. The privacy and darkness help decrease the amount of information from light, noise and other people to focus my energy back onto my future I have created and I am in love with.

With practice, I am able now to fill my body back up with the emotions of love, abundance, gratitude and worthiness. I become the creator of my life instead of the victim of it. But first, I have to catch myself in order not to get sucked into the old subconscious program. As I become conscious of what I am actually being, I get right back to feeling and being the elevated emotions of my future, which I am going to teach you how to create right now!

## Creating Your Future

Now comes the fun part. You are going to create the future you want! You are going to determine your target and recalibrate your body to feel this future before it becomes manifest in your life.

You might be asking, "Why did we not start with this step?" A very good question. The answer is that we have to know what the problem is in order to fix it. The previous step was designed to make us aware of what we may have once been unaware of. If 95% of our energy is being directed to subconscious activities in our body, then we need to pay attention to what is going on in our state of being the majority of the time. Only by observing ourself from a higher perspective, are we able to break the cycle of what has been subconsciously running our state of being. By doing this, we are disconnecting the old habitual synaptic connections in our brain, and by doing the work of this upcoming step, we are going to grow new synaptic brain connections to the future we dream of.

We are now aware of what we were once unaware because we have taken a good look at what kind of person we were being. This increase of awareness gives us the ability to catch ourselves getting sucked into the old programs. The minute we catch our-selves falling back into our old subconscious programs, we take our power back. We are free from the energetic burdens of all the negative emotions running us. We now have free energy to put to good use. The energy we would have used to hate our co-worker and continue down the emotional rabbit hole of judgement, hate and anger, is now available energy to be used in a much more productive manner. We can now choose (because we have become conscious of our state of being) to use the available energy to generate the feelings of our future we decide to create.

But first, you must get clear on what you want. It does not matter what you are doing. If you do not have a purpose, it is going to be impossible to accomplish anything. Think about it. Let us use the example of driving somewhere. Every time you get in your car, you know where you are going. You have a purpose. Your purpose is to get wherever you intended. The concept is, no doubt, very simple but the carrying out of the action is the challenge.

Just as you have a clear intention when you get in your car to go to the grocery store, you must create a clear intention when you want to achieve the desire of your dreams. Or simply to heal your pain and dysfunction of your body. Or to find the love of your life. It is the same formula for all manifestations whether it be reversing a dis-ease or buying your dream house.

Ask yourself questions like these:

What is the greatest version of myself I can be?

What would my dream life feel like?

How would I act if all my needs were met?

If I could be free to do whatever I want whenever I want, what would a typical day look like?

What people would I surround myself with?

How much money would I make and have in my bank account?

Who would I share my life with?

Where would I travel?

What adventures would I go on?

What is my purpose on this planet?

What will it feel like to be pain free?

What will it feel like to be disease free?

Find a quiet space and really spend some time with this and write down answers. Think big. Get real with yourself. Go within and focus your attention on what you really want and what life would be like without the pain or the dis-ease. This is hard to do because it requires you to become greater than your current level of consciousness. You must think greater than you currently feel. You have to start somewhere, but remember you have free energy to use from letting go of the emotions of your past. Just do it and as you practice it will undoubtedly become easier.

After this writing exercise, it is time now to get clear on how the new you will think, act, and feel, since this is what our personality is made up of. In our mind, we have to create a very clear model or image of what we want. This image, model or dream of the new you needs to be connected to a high vibrational emotion. An emotion of love, joy, awe, relief, abundance, wealth, peace, inspiration, etc. This image and emotion will motivate, inspire and come from within the truth of who you really are. It must light you up. You must establish the feeling within your body and connect deeply with it. Essentially, you must teach your body how this event will feel before it happens. When you have a clear image or intention of what you want, coalesced with a very high emotion of how it will feel when it comes to life, you are creating an energetic signature that the quantum field will respond to.

Answer these questions to begin to cultivate the new person you are going to create.

How will you think as the new you?

How will the new you think?

What kind of thoughts will the new you have?

What is your new attitude toward life going to be like?

How will you and others perceive the new you?

How will you act?

What are the moment-to-moment actions of the new you?

What will you do daily?

How will you communicate this new you to the world?

How will you live your life differently in this new energy?

How will you feel?

What amazing emotions will you become so familiar with that they become your new normal?

How will those emotions make you feel?

What kind of energy will you have on a moment-to-moment basis?

How will your body feel? Really learn to feel that feeling in your body.

## Putting It All Together

We will now build on the understanding of the role of epigenetics, psychoneuroimmunology and the quantum field that we learned earlier to examine how we can harness them in our creative process.

It should feel pretty good to have done the work of writing down who you have been, admitting and declaring it and then letting go. On the other side of the coin, it should create a great amount of joy, excitement and inspiration in your soul to have gotten clearer on who you want to be, how you want to act, and what things you will create in your life. This is where everything comes together and you can now understand a bit more of the mystical and how synchronicities, serendipities and healings actually happen.

We have been conditioned to believe it takes a struggle and a fight to get what we want in our life. We believe that in order to get the dream car, house, partner, job, vacation or whatever material thing we are striving for, we must drag our body to a job that we do not particularly care for in order to make enough money to be able to buy, afford or pay off what we want. There is nothing wrong with this. Do not get me wrong. It can work, but it is going to take a lot of time. In the same way, it means we think to heal our pain or disease that someone (doctor) or something (pharmaceutical drug or surgery) is going to heal our pain and fix us. We have been programmed to believe something outside us will fix the void inside us.

There is an alternative and much different way to create things and health in our life, though, and that is creating through the quantum realm. But to create through the invisible world of the quantum, we cannot be living in a scarcity mindset. We must literally believe we already have that desire in our possession. We have to live in that emotion it creates. We must be it, feel it and behave as if we already have it.

You see, when we are living in lack, we are usually not in our greatest version of ourself. The greatest version of ourself would be living as if we already possess that "thing" we want. In lack, we are wishing and wanting. We believe we are separate from that something out there that is going to make us happy. By thinking this outside "thing" will create our relief, we subconsciously believe we are separate from it. In other words, it is not in our possession yet. We believe the thing out there is going to fill some emotional void we need to fill. In doing this, we give all our power to the material possession, pill, surgery or person we think will make us whole again. This in turn takes away the available healing power we need. Likewise, it's the same power that brings material things we want into our life.

We all know the story of when we finally get our dream car or new pair of shoes we have wanted for so long. After about three months of driving the car or wearing the shoes, that feeling we were searching for by attaining that specific goal wears off. It is not the "thing" that is going to fill the void. By still believing it is the material thing, we are tricked again to think that we need something, someone or somewhere else material to make us happy.

It is an illusion that something else from the outside will fix whatever we are missing on the inside. And this materialistic, wishing and wanting cycle continues only to leave us wanting more. As you practice the above writing exercise and begin your daily meditation practice, you will see this from the inside. It will begin to make more sense as you become the master of your own emotions. You are the generator of these emotions all on your own. You hold the power, not them. When you realize this and sustain the energy of the future you have just created, the quantum law does the rest. All you are doing is changing your energetic signature of who you are being to which the field responds.

When we are living in the state of lack, we have learned through the new sciences we are creating chemical signatures of that state into our body. Our body then becomes chemically familiar with the energy that lack is creating. We become programmed below our awareness to be running in this state. All day long we are thinking and feeling, feeling and thinking that we need that new car, new job, new partner, new pill, etc. to give us the feeling of satisfaction and wholeness we so long for. Yet nothing new is happening in our life. It is like we are just running in place and getting nowhere. When we are separate from that feeling of actually having it, we continue to believe it is the something, someone or someplace outside of us that will bring us the joy, peace, relief, love, abundance, success, etc. We think that material thing will make us whole.

Living in this state has a certain vibration attached to it that we are transmitting to the quantum field. And now we understand that this state of being also has an energetic, chemical, hormonal and biochemical signature to the cells of our body. This signature has a direct effect on what genes are upregulated or downregulated in our body. In other words what genes are turned on and what genes are turned off directly effecting our health.

Remember how our car stereo picks up the vibrational match of the radio station that we tune our radio dial to? Well, this is exactly the same process of how we create things in our life too. When we are extremely clear on what we want and are able to generate the feelings of already having that thing, we are transmitting a very clear signal into the field. This clear signal starts to harmonize closer to the vibration of the thing we desire. Our desire is already a potential in the quantum field because all things exist in the field. When our frequency matches the frequency of the potential outcome in the field that we wish to manifest, whatever it may be, then we start to see evidence in our three-dimensional world. Things only we can know because they have a special meaning to us. We are literally getting feedback from the infinite intelligence of the divine. On the contrary, however, when we are stuck living in lack, hoping and wishing for that thing, our vibration and energy is not going to connect with the potential of it happening. Therefore, nothing new happens.

The important take away of this is that our state of being is not only influencing the health of our cells, but it is also influencing what we get or do not get in our reality. In other words, our state of being, which is how we think, feel and act, is either creating the life of our dreams or creating a life that we feel victim too.

Here is a scientific example of how by changing our state of being to one of love and joy we can create health in our body. Joe Dispenza and his team conducted a study on gratitude. They took 120 people in a week-long workshop and measured their cortisol and IgA (immunoglobulin A) levels. As we have previously learned, cortisol is a stress hormone, and when we are living under the dominance of the sympathetic nervous system, cortisol levels are very high. IgA is a protein that is part of our amazing immune system. IgA has been shown by science to be one of the strongest immune system defenses against bacteria, toxins and other chemicals that invade the body. IgA is created automatically by our body, and it is very strong and essential in keeping us alive. When cortisol goes up, IgA goes down, and the converse is also true. When IgA is up, cortisol is down. This means that when IgA is down and stress is up, we are more prone to disease.

The study asked these 120 people to spend 9-10 minutes three times a day in a state of gratitude, joy and love. The study aimed to show that elevated states of emotions would increase the IgA levels in the body and decrease cortisol. The results of the study confirmed just that. It showed that the cortisol levels of the participants went down three standard deviations from their normal, and their IgA levels raised on an average of 52.5 to 86 mg/DL.

What this means is that by changing our state of being we not only have the capability to dramatically improve our health, but we also have the ability to reverse pain and disease. If we can increase the strongest immune fighter we know of by simply feeling the state of joy, gratitude and love three times a day, 10 minutes at a time, then imagine what other health promoting genes we can, epigenetically, regulate upward.

By doing the above exercise and beginning your daily meditation practice, you will no longer be as easily sucked into the old habitual states of anger, fear, unworthiness, etc. that you used to. As you practice unlearning these emotions by becoming aware of how they have been running your unconscious program, you will lose the emotional charge they previously had on your body. Every time you catch these emotions before they take root and run an old program, you will unwire the neural connection in your brain. This will turn the unwanted old habit into wisdom. Wisdom is simply a memory without an emotion connected to it. Wisdom allows you to see the past at a higher state of consciousness. It simply no longer affects you.

As you unlearn and unwire the neural connections in your brain from your past emotions, you replace it with the new connection and wiring of new heart-based emotion. The emotions of gratitude, joy, abundance, worthiness, wealth, health, freedom, etc. with practice feeling and thinking, thinking and feeling these heart-based emotions, you will sprout and grow new neural pathways in the brain. According to Hebb's law, neurons that fire together wire together, and conversely, nerves that unwire no longer fire together. This is what you are creating in your brain as you keep practicing.

In Hebb's law, nerves that continually fire and wire together grow stronger electrical charges. This is why habitual thoughts are so hard to break, because they have a deeper-rooted electrical charge. I like to think of Hebb's law as the Grand Canyon. As the water flows continually over the same rock, it wears deep into the earth creating a canyon. Similarly, the nerves become entrained with the same wiring as habitual thoughts are fired recurrently, creating a deep pathway of electrical flow in the brain. The good news is Hebb's Law also states that when nerves no longer fire and wire together, their strength diminishes. This means that as we catch ourselves getting pulled into our old thought patterns of guilt, shame, unworthiness, anger, frustration, jealousy, etc. and choose to stop thinking that way, we begin to disconnect the strong deep-rooted connections.

The triggers that used to annoy you or anger you integrate, and you will no longer be sucked into that habit. You will find you are greater than that, and you know the old habit has an epigenetic signature in your body that created problems. You now understand you would never want to hurt yourself like that. Being a victim, blaming, hating or getting angry at someone, something or someplace is only hurting you, diminishing the energetic vibration being sent into the field and overburdening your body with the stress hormones.

But now as you practice the new you and who that person will be, how she will act and how she will think, you can insert that new personality into your daily life. You no longer will be annoyed and judging your co-worker because you will be captivated by the emotional signature of the personality you are now being. You will be consumed by the future you are creating and not want to give the incredible energy of it away to someone, something or somewhere else.

As you become the new you, you are electromagnetically transmitting an entirely new vibration into the quantum field. Eastern medicine has known for thousands of years that the human body is a magnet and has an electromagnetic field around it—just as the earth does. In western medicine, however, very little validity is given to the importance of how coherent or incoherent the electromagnetic field of our entire body is. Even though in conventional ways, we use things like a magnetic resonance imaging (MRI) machine to measure the amount of magnetic fields and radio waves we emit to better image the tissues of our body.

Nonetheless, we now have a greater consciousness, knowing the more coherent and orderly our electromagnetic field is around our body, the better our cells function. Popp showed this in his work with biophotons and their light emittance. Just because we cannot see it does not mean this energy does not exist. Our heart, too, has its own electromagnetic field that has been measured in a distance up to nine feet in all directions of our body, i.e., a circle with its center in the body and a radius of nine feet. More on the astonishing heart in Section Three.

When we are living in our new personality with a clear intention and an elevated emotion, we are sending out a much stronger signal into the field. Not only does this elevated thought and feeling combination produce the biochemistry in our body to promote homeostasis, repair and regeneration, it also sends a much more rhythmic and orderly signal into the field. Our clear intention or thought is responsible for the signal sent out into the field and our elevated heart-felt emotion is what draws the energy back to us. This synchronized energy we have created makes a torus field around our bodies. The heart also has its own toric field which we will discuss in more detail in the next section.

We are now vibrating in a very rhythmic, orderly fashion, and when this happens all our energy centers are in a better alignment. Each energy center, or chakra as the ancient yogic tradition has named them, has a little mind and energy of its own. When the energy centers are running with better coherence and energy, the cells in the tissues function much better. (We will go into much more detail of the energy centers in Section Three.) In this state, we have an orderly and coherent energy running through us and all around us. This is our energetic body.

Remember the visible light spectrum that is less than 1% of what we have found to be in the field? There is energy and information within us and all around us, always. When we match our energetic field with a possibility that is already in this infinite energy that is always around us, our desire manifests in 3D reality.

Here is an example of how this happens. When two acoustic guitars are side by side and you pluck a G string of one guitar, the other guitar's G string magically starts to play. How does this happen? It happens because of the quantum field of energy and information all around us. The invisible field is full of information in it that connects the two strings. Just as you are already connected to your desired future outcome. When there is a vibrational match in the field more order is created. More energy is created. Because the two G strings have and equal vibration and energy, they match, and the G string that was plucked starts to resonate with the energy in the field, causing the other G string of the guitar to play without being touched.

This is exactly what happens in our life when we start to become our new personality. We are emitting a different energy and vibration into the field, a much stronger and more coherent energy at that. We notice random and unplanned things will start to happen in our lives equal to that vibration. Little signs that create awe. New opportunities and synchronicities arise. No matter how small or big they may seem, these are extremely important signs that we are connecting to our new energy we desire to manifest. Our internal state is creating external things to show up in our life. These signs are very personal to us. Only we can know them. We now have evidence we are the creators of our own destiny.

We will not be able to predict this event, because if we can, then we know it. If we know it, then we are back to predicting or anticipating. When we are in the state of anticipation, we are trying to control. And this lowers our vibrational signature. There is no longer a match to the desired outcome we have been working on.

The quantum field does not work in an anticipatory fashion. The quantum field works in an unpredictable, individual to you, knock your socks off, unbelievable but trusting kind of way. Whatever our desired event is will come to us in a way we cannot predict.

Just like we did not even think about a phone call from our mom would simultaneously happen while we were thinking of her. Or a time in your life where something worked out in just the right time for you to achieve your goal. Or perhaps a time when you were thinking a thought of a specific thing or symbol, and then moments later, this very same symbol or thing shows up in your three-dimensional reality. This synchronistic event is only plausible to you. Our desire will come in a way we least expect. This is how the governing consciousness works.

## Quick Takeaways From Stress

1. We experience stress anytime our brain and body get knocked out of balance because of a perceived threat.

2. In today's world, this is mostly from thought alone.

3. In stress, we do not digest food optimally – over time this alone causes many diseases.

4. The ego wants us to stay the same because it is familiar.

5. The ego makes us think the unknown (change) will kill us. The ego literally tricks us to believe this change could actually kill us.

6. It will not kill us.

7. We have to know what the problem is in order to change or fix it.

8. We have to spend time observing that problem, which means we must observe how we have been being, acting and behaving.

9. Awareness is key, because once we are so vigilantly aware of our thoughts and feelings, we would never choose to think the old programmed thoughts.

10. Now we create our future by getting very clear on who we want to be and what we want to experience as far as feelings and emotions from our new self.

11. Our old self (lower vibrational emotions) creates disease. Our new self (higher vibrational emotions) creates health through epigenetics and psychoneuroimmunology.

# Meditation

In the area of meditation techniques, I have based my personal practice on the work of Joe Dispenza. You will find the reference to his work in the Further Reading section. However, it is important for you to find the style of meditation that is most comfortable for you. By now you should have learned that to take your power back you must first do what speaks to you innately. My goal in this section is to help you understand that you *can* meditate with ease. You do not have to live on the top of a mountain in a Buddhist monastery to meditate. You will learn by gaining this knowledge that you are able to tap into this state anywhere.

Meditation simply means to awaken yourself or, in other words, to get to know yourself. In the Tibetan culture, the meditation symbol means to become familiar with. Meditation is the best and most readily accessible tool to get to know who we truly are. This is because, through meditation, we are entering into the subconscious mind. Remember that 95% of our total energy is used in the subconscious and only 5% being our conscious mind. It is estimated that the subconscious mind is processing 4,000,000,000 bits of information per second compared to the conscious mind's 2,000. This means the subconscious is two million times faster than the conscious mind. It is obvious that if we want to find out who we truly are and tap into our innate power within, we have to enter into our subconscious mind.

Within our subconscious is a knowing of our higher self that is much deeper than our name, our occupation or where we are from. This knowing is on a soul level. The parts of ourselves we cannot see; that in which brings all life in our 3D world into existence. Remember that all the previous work above of self-reflection and creating your future self is done to prepare you to create this state of being in your daily meditation.

As we get out of our analytical mind through meditation, we strip away the layers of our ego, allowing our true divinity to raise to our awareness. When we get a taste of this, we no longer want to take part in anything other than greatness. At this point we become infatuated because we have a deep connection to this remembering of a very familiar yet hard to put into words kind of enlightenment.

## Our Analytical Mind

From the moment we start to wake from our sleep, the mind starts to analyze all the things going on in our life. From what we are going to wear to what we are going to make for dinner to what so and so is doing on Facebook. We get stuck in the world of our senses. What we can see, taste, smell, hear and touch. Whatever it may be that the five senses bring us, our mind is constantly analyzing it.

When our analytical mind is running, our brain is emitting beta brain waves into the field. Brainwaves are electrical impulses the brain emits into the field all around us as the mind is working its magic. Scientists, medical professionals, and even the lay person can measure these brainwaves by using a device called an electroencephalography (EEG). This amazing tool tells us what electrical impulses the brain is emitting. Below are images of the five brainwave states we can be in.

# HUMAN BRAIN WAVES

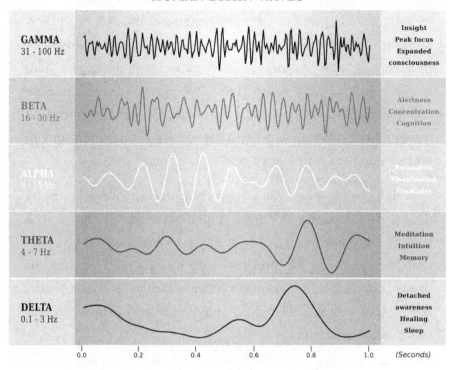

| | | |
|---|---|---|
| **GAMMA** 31 - 100 Hz | | Insight Peak focus Expanded consciousness |
| **BETA** 16 - 30 Hz | | Alertness Concentration Cognition |
| **ALPHA** 8 - 15 Hz | | Relaxation Visualization Creativity |
| **THETA** 4 - 7 Hz | | Meditation Intuition Memory |
| **DELTA** 0.1 - 3 Hz | | Detached awareness Healing Sleep |

0.0     0.2     0.4     0.6     0.8     1.0     (Seconds)

*Figure 5*

In the beta brainwave state, we are in our conscious mind. We are focusing on the external environment and the analyzation of it. Our mind has a tremendous amount of dispersed energy happening in it as the different areas of the brain are all firing and wiring to process the many things we are focusing on in our outer environment. For example, during a conversation with another person, our brain is likely in high beta where it is processing everything the other person is saying and formulating the reply we want to give.

As the brainwaves slow in frequency, they move into a lower beta. We are likely in low beta when we are relaxed and reading a book or listening to a lecture. This is all still the analytical mind. However, in low beta the brainwaves slow down a bit as we are analyzing what we are receiving from our senses and formulating our own understanding of it. When the brainwave's frequency slows even more, we go from low beta into alpha. This is where there is a blurry line, unique to every individual person, where we slip into our subconscious mind. We are no longer analyzing all the different outside components of our environment, and we enter into our inner world of the dream state.

Think back to when you were a child, and you played and day dreamed all day long. When you put a broom stick between your legs, and in your mind, it was really a rocket ship. Or you pretended to be a dog for the entire day, using an old box as your doggy bed. This is the subconscious mind, and children under the age of seven years old live in it. They have very little analytical mind. They believe in everything.

Meditation helps us get out of our analytical mind and into our subconscious mind. The world we live in keeps us stuck in our analytical mind. Children have the joy of escaping and dreaming a world of thoughts and things into reality. Why do you think they are so happy? And do not see skin color? Or social status? They are not analyzing every little detail to the finest T. They couldn't care less. Thus, we see their default state is joy and happiness.

In order to truly change, we have to change the old habitual programs that have been running subconsciously. Meditation is hands down the best tool to reprogram our subconscious habits from old to new. Not only does it start to generate the new personality by bringing us the elevated emotions of it, but it breaks us away from our old habitual self. We have to break the ties keeping us stuck in the box of our current reality. During meditation, when we get out of our analytical mind and enter into the truth of who we really are, we are cutting the cords that keep us stuck. We are teaching our mind and body how to feel relief, peace and bliss.

The act of meditating reroutes the flow of energy constantly being used to run our over-analytical mind. This is a relief to our body and nervous system, allowing it to have the energy it needs to do what it is supposed to do naturally. Not only are we able to hear the story of our soul through our subconscious mind giving us great insight, but we learn to quiet our analytical mind so we are able to loosen its grip on us in our daily lives. This gives us our power back. There is an elegant connection to all of life in our subconscious mind. Meditation rekindles this flame.

As we enter our subconscious through a meditative process, our muscles relax. Our body lets go. We start to feel relief. Our mind is slowing its brainwaves down into the alpha state. Here we are free from the stresses of our busy life. Consequently, we are regenerating our body through epigenetics and psychoneuroimmunology.

Somewhere between alpha and theta is the sweet spot of timelessness. This is where we enter the quantum field—the field where everything is possible, where there are no limits. There is no time. Where you are not your body, your name, your race or your gender. This is the land of oneness and unity. Without things, there is just eternal blackness. You are only your consciousness.

## The Present Moment–Eternal Now of The Quantum Field

To be in the present moment, you cannot be recalling, analyzing or reliving old memories. Equally, you cannot be in the future trying to predict, control or manipulate some future outcome. The present moment can only be right now in a space that is eternal. Eternal means there is an infinite duration, and because we are so used to time being linear, eternity is a difficult concept for us to grasp.

When we get past our analytical mind running the show, we gracefully fall into the present moment. In this moment is eternity because there is no time as we know it. This is the fifth dimension of the quantum world. In the quantum, all possibilities exist, and we do not have to travel through space to get to them. Whatever our intention is we can receive. But this is tricky because in the quantum there are no things. It is vast nothingness. So, in the present moment we are beyond our body. And we are beyond our identity. We are no longer associating reality with our senses. Therefore, we practice meditation, eliminating any chance of our five senses being stimulated. The elimination of the five senses distracting us allows us to get to the present moment without being tapped back into our five senses.

If we associate with our desire by feeling the lack of not having it, we cannot be in the present moment. This is because we have just made it separate from us by thinking I want this thing, but I do not have it yet. We believe it is separate from our possession. In the present moment, however, we already have it, because in this dimension, there is no separation. It is a vacuum of a single point. The tiniest point of singularity. And what is singularity? Well, it is whole. Everything is in union. And nothing is separate, so that means *you* are it.

This is extremely weird, I know. But as you practice putting your awareness on the present moment in meditation, you begin to develop the neural connections to feel and embody this truth. Words cannot describe this, so again, you just have to do it, working through the games of your ego trying to talk you out of it. With practice, like anything else, meditation becomes more familiar to you.

In this space of the present moment, you do not have to try or seek because it is already there. Remember it is not separate from you. This creates a feeling of pure relief and bliss. We feel safe, whole and complete because we already have it. Nothing is missing. Our body, in which we are still conscious of but not really in it, gets an upgrade of not needing anything because we already have everything. The word I use to describe this is relief. In the present moment, I personally feel the peace of having relief.

So, pause for a moment, right now, and imagine you already have that thing which you are seeking. Take a moment and feel that you have it. By doing this exercise and aligning your mind and body in the same intention, your body just felt, physiologically, that you have it. This is because the body is objective, and it does not know the difference between actually having "the thing" or the belief of having it.

As we practice using the following meditation techniques and letting go, we learn to simply *BE* in the present moment. We realize we are love, and that is where we have come from. Our ego no longer has as tight a grip on us, and we begin to feel empowered and worthy to receive all the gifts we have been conditioned to think we need. Remember these gifts do not come as things. (Although, as you practice being in this present moment, they might show up as things in your life.) They come to us as a feeling or a consciousness. For it is merely the feeling we are searching for when we think a particular thing is going to bring us happiness. Instead of being so concerned with "things," we now realize we already have what we are longing for.

The present moment happens when our consciousness becomes one or merges with the collective consciousness, which is the quantum field. There is a unification process that happens. We simply connect with what truly is. And remember what truly is the quantum field is an invisible field of infinite possibilities all around us. By eliminating the stimulation of our five senses and entering the blackness, we tap into the infinite intelligence that is the soup of the quantum. This creates amazing feelings of transcendence into our being. These elevated feelings of transcendence let us know we are there.

As we continue to feel these heightened states of bliss during our meditation practice, we know we are becoming more and more singularity. We are becoming more and more whole. Total oneness. Here is the present moment, and we receive everything, we become everyone, we are everywhere and we are in every time. We have to be because we have become singularity.

Every night as we drift away to sleep, we go from beta to alpha to theta to delta. While sleeping, we go through all the processes of sleep, like REM and deep sleep. Thanks to science, we have been able to associate these different processes of sleep to respective brainwave states. Sleep is an unconscious phenomenon, and our body automatically does this every night. We just let go. My point is we know how to do this already. We know how to let go because we do it every night. Keep in mind that when we practice meditation, we are doing the same thing except we remain conscious instead of falling into the sleep state. With practice, we become aware of how to fall into the space just before we drift off into the unconscious sleep state. As we continue to practice, we can tell if we are in alpha or not. We learn to know if we are over analyzing or not.

A helpful tip—when meditating in your chair, if your head starts to bob like you are drifting away to sleep, this is a good sign you are entering the alpha brainwave state. Do not worry because your neck will learn to brace itself as you meditate more and more.

Before long, you will know by the feeling you get if you are there in alpha or not.

This carries over into our daily life, and we are now more aware that we are in analysis paralysis. Analysis paralysis is a play on words because we get sucked back into our old programs and go down the rabbit hole of an old habitual state of being. The over analysis causes us to almost be paralyzed from realizing it. But with a daily meditation practice, we are teaching our brain and body how it feels to be out of the over-analytical state, so we can be more aware during our day when it sucks us back in unconsciously.

There is nothing wrong with analyzing. We must do it to stay alive. But again, it's about a balance. We have to learn to understand when we are in a state of fear and over analyzing or in a state of love and trusting in the Divine intelligence within us and all around us. As we practice meditating, we learn how to let go and trust in the intelligence that is creating all of life. We simply stop trying and start to trust that thy will be done. When we are trusting in the intelligence taking care of everything we could ever need, there is no more reason to analyze because we know it will happen in the way it is supposed to.

We begin to find ourselves when we get out of our own way. When we start to get out of our own way, our brainwaves slow down into the alpha, theta and delta brainwave states. Our brain becomes more rhythmic and orderly, synchronizing together. When we do this, we are not analyzing. We let go. We surrender and trust, trust and surrender. The infinite intelligence within us and all around us is able to take over. It begins to create order in our biology. It gives us insights in our mind's eye. It calms us down into the parasympathetic nervous system. It helps us see things from a higher perspective (a different point of view). After we get up from our meditation, we are a different person than when we sat down.

## Preparation

It is imperative to have a dark and quiet room or space to meditate in. If you have children, prepare to have someone else watch them or let them know this is your time, and they are not to bother you unless in an emergency. Use a comfortable chair or pillow to sit on so you are in an upright, seated posture. I like to use a blindfold to keep even more light out from distracting my brain to create total blackness. I also cover up with a blanket during my morning meditations to create the most comfortable environment in order for my body to relax. Try not to have anything cooking or coffee being made to ensure you are not stimulating your sense of smell. Put your phone on silent or airplane mode if you have music downloaded to your phone. Headphones with soft meditative music playing provide a great way to keep any surrounding noises from distracting your focus. Plus, much of the meditation music available has a calming frequency as its undertone. You can search for meditation music on YouTube, Spotify or Apple music. There are thousands of tracks. Find a 30-minute to one-hour song that resonates with you. If you are beginning, use this same song every meditation as your brain will associate it with the alpha, theta and delta brainwave state.

As you can see, you want to eliminate all the five senses in order to quiet your brain from stimulation. When it is not having to pick up any external senses, it is primed and ready to become coherent and drift away into alpha.

## Meditation Techniques

The following forms of meditation are simply ways to get your brain and body to work in a more coherent and orderly fashion. By focusing on one thing, your brain slows down from high beta and calms its sporadic firing all throughout the brain to come into alignment and attunement. As it focuses on a single thing, it cannot be so disorderly firing in all directions. It is just as a flock of starlings fly together in unity, where thousands of birds look like one whole organism. As you train your brain and body in meditation, it will come together in harmony like we see in all nature.

## The Breath Meditation

Probably the most common form of meditation is the practice of following your breath. After all, it is the breath that brings us to life. When it stops, our soul leaves our body. We cannot see the air in which we breathe, but the air's invisible essence gives life to our body. Consequently, the breath is the miracle between the invisible world of the governing consciousness behind all material things and our material body. It is the connection between mind and body. Mind being the invisible quantum world and body being the manifestation of the mind into the material. The breath is the essence that connects both worlds.

There is no right or wrong way to follow your breath. The breath is remarkable because it is never unavailable for us to tap into. It is always there. Remember the whole point is to have your brain focus on one task, in this case your breath, so that it is not sporadically firing in different regions. This is what we are aiming for in meditation, as this is the key to slip into the subconscious and let go of the tight grip of the controlling and anticipatory nature of the analytical mind.

Let us start with a victory. I like to teach this meditation first in order to prove to my patients/clients that they *can* meditate.

I call it, "Take Three." To start, sit in a comfortable chair in a dark room, set your timer on your phone for three minutes and turn on your soft meditation music. Close your eyes and breathe in through your nose for four seconds and breathe out through your nose for four seconds. Repeat this until the timer sounds.

See how you feel. Did you relax? Do you feel less tense? Did three minutes feel like an hour? Congratulations, you have just meditated!

Check in with yourself and take inventory of your state. If you want more, use this same technique but set timer for five or more minutes. Continue daily.

## Diaphragmatic Breathing

In the breath comes a multifaceted number of benefits, enough to write hundreds of books on the topic. But to help you better understand the power of your breath, I want to introduce you to one of its very powerful capabilities. As you know, when you breathe deeply, which we all have done, there is a relaxing nature to it. This powerful aspect alone must be taken advantage of to calm ourselves from the stressed (fight or flight) state of being to the calm and relaxed (rest and digest) state of being. More specifically, when we breathe deeply into our belly, using our diaphragm, we are undoubtedly switching into the rest and digest (parasympathetic) nervous system. This is a powerful tool.

To do this, sit or lay down on your back and get comfortable. First, breathe in through your nose, keeping your mouth closed and your tongue lightly pressed on the backside of your upper teeth. This aligns your jaw to allow maximum oxygen into and through the airway. On the inhalation, take a big deep breath in and feel the air come into your chest, then down into your belly. As the air comes in, allow your belly to expand like a balloon. You may place your hand on your belly just over your naval to give you feedback of this action. Breathe in for four seconds, and exhale for six seconds again out of your nose. As you exhale, be conscious of your belly collapsing back in like a balloon releasing the air inside it. This balloon contraction and expansion is the diaphragm muscle doing what it does.

Try this 10 times. You will feel totally relaxed after doing this compared to when you started. Do this throughout your day to take your power back and escape from the analytical mind.

## Box Breathing

Do not worry about breathing from your nose or mouth on this one. Refer to the Nike slogan and just do it!

1.  Breathe in for four seconds.

2.  Hold your breath for four seconds.

3.  Exhale slowly for four seconds.

4.  Pause after exhale for four seconds before inhaling.

Repeat this for 10 repetitions. You can now understand why it has been called the box breath. If four seconds is too short, add as many seconds as you can handle equally throughout the box breath. This technique is always available to you. Always!

An aside. Many people I work with tell me "there's no way I can meditate because I cannot stop my brain from thinking. It is just impossible for me." Hopefully you see by now that you are not stopping your brain from thinking, you are merely giving it another task while removing other stimuli. Your brain is going to start thinking about random things like what you are going to eat when you get up from your meditation. This is because you have conditioned your brain and body to do so. This is not a bad thing. It is simply what the brain and body are familiar with. Understand that your body is going to try to tell you to get up and see what that sound was. Or scratch the itch on your ear. Or go start the coffee maker. This is ok. It is part of the process. However...

It is your job to be aware of this and be the master of your mind and body by using your free will to get your mind back on track. Every time you come back to your breath, heart, mantra or divergent or convergent focus you have made a huge victory. Because every time you do this, you are coming back to the present moment instead of analyzing the past or the future. You bring your attention back to the present by following one of these techniques. This is creating the new neural networks in your brain to unseat the old habitual programs from running. Some days are harder than others. Some days are amazing and some days you have to work really hard to stay focused. But those hard days are the biggest wins because you are training your brain not to go into the old programs during your waking day.

## Mantra Meditation

The word mantra can be broken into two parts—"man" meaning mind and "tra" meaning a vehicle or transport. A mantra takes the form of sounds, words or vibrations repeated silently in your mind to transport you into a deep state of meditation. In transcendental meditation courses, a mantra is given to you by your teacher, but you do not have to be given a mantra by a teacher. You can create your own.

For example, I found it most helpful to have a mantra that was only sounds and meant absolutely nothing to me. However, some meditators like to use inspirational phrases like "I am strong" or "I am worthy" repeated. I have found that certain rhythmic sounds with no meaning associated in my mind, worked best for me to slip into the alpha brainwave state. Remember the whole point of a mantra is to occupy your mind on the mantra in order to quiet the rest of the mind chatter.

I used the sounds of Ah Lum BAR Dee Dum and then Ah Lum BAH Dee Dum repeated. This has an alternating BAR and then BAH to create a rhythmic tone to keep my mind from going into the random thoughts it normally would in the beta state. Another one I have heard used is Sha RING, Sha RING over and over.

After repeating this mantra, you will find that you slip away into a very relaxed meditative state and forget everything in your 3D world. After some time of silently repeating this mantra, you will be so relaxed you have forgotten about repeating it.

If you find this form of meditation works for you, practice for 15 to 20 minutes a day for three months. As you practice, you will become so familiar with it you will be able to do it automatically.

I have found that sometimes I like to have quiet music in my headphones, and sometimes I like pure silence. Only you know what is best.

## Heart Resonance Meditation

Step one—Put all your attention on and in the area of your heart. Focus on your breath going in and out of your heart space. It may help to place your hand on your heart to give your body feedback on this area.

Step two—While focusing your attention and breath in and on your heart space behind your sternum, bring up an elevated emotion such as love, gratitude, abundance, wholeness, worthiness, joy, bliss, a love for life. It helps to use someone or something you love in this world to spark this emotion. You can use the version of yourself you created earlier and generate the feeling you will get when this new you is manifested. Or what it will be like to receive the wealth, new job or partner you are longing for. Maybe your children, pet, mom, dad, brother, sister, uncle, or aunt. A scenic mountain view or a beach. Anything that generates this emotion will do. It's all about the feeling, not the material thing.

With practice, this emotion of love will grow and grow. Before long you will be able to tap into this emotion at will without needing any material thing or person to help you get into that emotion.

Inspirational meditative music is also a nice tool. Again, using the same song every time to give your brain a reminder. If this resonates with you, do it. Practice. If you are just beginning, start with five minutes and increase the time of your meditation as you improve.

## Convergent and Divergent Focus Meditation

To converge means to meet at a point. To diverge means to go in a different direction. Therefore, a convergent focus would be on a specific thing, and in meditation, we often use different parts or spaces in and on our body. A divergent focus would be to broaden your focus or see from a higher perspective. In meditation, we become aware of the space around our body, the space in the room that we are sitting, the space over and around the town we live in, and the space around the earth we live on. If we relate this to the quantum model of the particle and the wave, the convergent focus would be the manifestation of the particle, and the divergent focus would be the entire potential of the wave in the field around us.

Meditation is all about focus, and with focus we gain self-awareness. When we are more self-aware, we have choice of what we would like to focus on. This is how we raise our consciousness. Thicht Naht Han said, "Meditation is not a passive sitting in silence. It is a sitting in awareness, free from distraction, and realizing the clear understanding that arises from concentration." In meditation, when we practice changing our focus from our body (convergent) to the space around our body (divergent), we are practicing to control our awareness. The practice of this builds neural networks in our brain and body so we are more aware of where our attention and energy is going during the day when we are not meditating.

I find it works best to start with a convergent focus like the above increasing your heart's energy field meditation and gradually working divergently to feel the space around your heart. This is what we will learn in the next section as we place our attention first convergently on and then divergently around the energy centers of our body. As you practice, you will naturally start to feel the energy around the bodily energy center itself. This is the divergent focus and you will feel this because these powerful energetic centers of the body are emitting a field around them.

In this chakra awakening meditation that we will learn step-by-step at the end of the next section, you will start by placing your energy convergently on the first energy center of the perineum. You will keep your focused attention on this area in your body for a couple minutes and then feel the space divergently around your hips, which is the field or wave form of this center. From the first center of the perineum, you will then take your attention to the second center of the digestive hormonal center. And repeat the same process all the way to the eighth center above your head. The eighth center is by default a divergent focus as this center is not a part of the physical body. Likewise, as we build from the first energy center at the base of our spine up to the eighth energy center on top of our head, we will naturally feel the energy around our body in a divergent fashion.

Our natural state is unconditional love. Through meditation, as you get the analytical mind out of the way, the ego will quiet, and naturally, you will start to feel this love coming to the surface like a beach ball submerged in water. Not to mention, as you practice meditation, you become more self-aware of what the ego has been tricking you into believing as you constantly catch it throwing a fit for you to get up and do something. The combination of this awakening allows the unconditional love to rise to the surface of your awareness. Your true self. By default, as you quiet your analytical mind, you will feel more and more of the indescribable feelings of love, ecstasy, abundance, worthiness, brain and heart coherence, etc.

As you reach these states of elevated emotions and your body becomes more accustomed to them, you develop a new personality. This is the future you that already exists in the now. Feeling the elegant and blissful feelings that meditation creates, you will begin to look forward to meditating every day. This is not only because of the blissful feelings it creates during and after the act of meditation, but it is also because new opportunities and serendipities will show up in your life. These little signs from the universe create even more elevated emotions of inspiration and awe. These signs are guidance from the universe and will spark you to go even deeper and further to feel even more amounts of love, joy and bliss. Stay awake to these signs as the littlest things that have a deep meaning to you are huge signs you are connected to the Divine. These are a great guidance system to let you know you are on track and in the right state of being.

The challenge is to keep this elevated state you develop in your daily meditation all day long. This is the hard part. This means that when someone cuts you off in traffic, you must remember the elevated state you will feel when you have your dream life and not fall back into the old you and yell profanities. When you fall out of this elevated state, you are no longer a vibrational match to your new life. But do not worry because it's ok to experience these emotions since they are part of the human experience, but resilience is the key. You simply keep going and catch all the triggers in your life. Because, let us be honest, you are going to fall back into the old programs once in a while and react with judgement, blame or hate. That is ok. But staying in that low energy emotion for the rest of your day is not going to bring you the dream life you have created. It is all about bouncing back.

The more aware you are when this happens and the faster you bounce back are the keys. As you practice resilience and bounce back to your elevated state that connects you to your new life and future self, you will develop stronger neural networks for this. :ike building muscle in the gym, you will build pathways in the brain to make this a state of being and a habit. Likewise, every time you catch yourself reacting to the conditions in your life that cause you to judge, blame or hate and bounce back to your elevated state, you will unwire the old habitual low-energy stress neural networks. As we know from Hebb's Law, when we stop firing and wiring neurons, they no longer have a deep foothold in our brain. This means they will disappear.

In each of these forms of meditation I have gone through, you can choose if you would like to do them with guided help from a facilitator or on your own. For guided help, search the Internet for guided breath meditations or guided meditations.

Meditation is the key that unlocks the change we have been longing for. It allows us to have the feelings of whatever it is we are tricked into thinking is going to make us happy. We are literally feeling as if we already have it. As we practice our daily meditation, we realize we really do not need anything because we already have it. We become so good at feeling the emotions we have so longed to have from receiving some thing, some relationship, some job or some place that we no longer want it. Because we are so fulfilled, we are whole. Thus, we let go, trust and feel our intuition that is guided by the power of the universe.

We are now equipped with a powerful tool to awaken our truest self daily. In the moment of our meditation when we feel the indescribable feelings of love, gratitude, wholeness and oneness, it is our job to remember this feeling and embody it into every cell. After our meditation, we must intently focus on remembering this feeling throughout our entire day. The more we are in this state during our day, the more amazing circumstances will show up in our 3D life.

## A Victim State of Being

With the ever-available information we have at our fingertips, there is a lot of talk about the victim mindset. I have already mentioned it a couple of times, but I want to make sure we unravel what it truly means to be a victim of our reality or the creator of it.

If someone, something, some place, or some experience in your life causes you to change your internal state, then you are a victim of that circumstance. For instance, if I ask you how you are doing today, and you tell me, "Well, I was doing really well until some crazy driver cut me off, speeding down the freeway, so now I am very angry because he could have killed me!" You are now a victim of that circumstance as it altered your internal state of being.

This is mostly happening subconsciously. We are constantly being frustrated, angered or annoyed by some person (mostly people) some place or something. These happenings in our external environment are changing our state of being internally. We blame the person for our bad day or our frustration. In our conscious mind, it is their fault. Not ours. This is being a victim. *THEY* are controlling how *WE* feel inside.

When we do this, we are giving our internal lifeforce energy away to that circumstance. As we have learned, where we place our attention is where we place our energy. And because of this person we think is the problem, we now are giving all of our energy away to them. Instead of being in control of where it goes.

This is not a bad thing. And as I have said before it is going to happen, but the whole key again is awareness that we are doing it. It is very tricky to catch because most of us have done this our whole lives without even knowing it.

What is truly phenomenal, though, is that we can learn to regulate this. This is self-regulation. With a daily meditation practice and taking what we are learning about ourselves from the meditation, we become more aware of what is going on in our internal state of being during the day. We start to become conscious of what we were once unconscious of, awakening us to make a change in our state of being for the better. In doing this, we can regulate our energy distribution. We understand we are in control of where our energy is going. We realize, "Geez, why would I want to give my power away to something outside of me that I cannot control?" We catch ourselves slipping and draw our energy back.

What is even more phenomenal is that things in our outer world start to change. We start to see a change in our three-dimensional world all because we have changed our internal state. These are the coincidences, synchronicities, serendipities and new opportunities we just spoke of that give us inspiration that we are on the right path. They reassure us we are actually making internal changes. Because we are changing our internal state by becoming more aware of where our energy/power is going, we have more energy available for our cells to work with as our freewill brings our attention back to our body.

## Power of Saying No

Our truth and innate wisdom evolve naturally as we have taken the previous steps to become aware of who we were being and created a clear picture of who we want to be. It is not some convoluted scheme you can buy from an Instagram influencer. Nobody or nothing is going to do it for you. It comes built in and preassembled, but we have to connect with it. In the most subtle way, as we start to live our truth and awaken, we are going to say no to things we do not want to do. Previously in our lives, we have agreed to do many things we did not want to do. We may have or may have not been able to feel our intuition speaking to us on a soulful level. Innocently agreeing to things that really did not feel right or that we really did not want to do just to appease others. I do not know about you, but I used to do this all the time. I was consistently doing things so others did not perceive me the wrong way. The act of these minor decisions over time creates a major incongruence in our biology. It does not match our true self. And as you know, when things do not match, they create dis-ease in our body.

Our deep gut level is now awakened (further details on how to in the next section), and we will listen to it. Think of all the times you wanted to say no, but some other person or thing influenced you from saying no. When we are not in alignment with our truth and we do things for others only to look good, we are giving our innate healing power away. This is our choice, but as we become clear on our truth, naturally, we take our power back and say no to the things we want to. In doing so, you will now be aware of any guilt, shame or feeling bad for hurting someone else's feelings. You now know you are going to take your power back.

## The Power of Saying Yes

Not only will you have the rooted foundation to say no without guilt, the same thing goes for saying yes. Now that you know the difference between who you want to be and who you do not want to be, you can say yes to your yes. To say this another way, you now have created more awareness to do more of what you want to do. You are now clear on what you want. To take action, you simply stay in alignment with what you want. This makes yes and no's very natural. Conversely, it makes saying no much easier because you have woken up to the fact that you may have been doing things not in alignment with who you truly are.

To be clear, I am not saying that you should go and quit your job as soon as possible. This means you can now make little adjustments in your day-to-day decisions to take your power back. Each decision being in better alignment with who you truly are is a victory. With time and your daily meditation practice, you will be in total alignment with the truth of who you really are. You will feel your energy increase as your actions match your truth. Your heart will open wide and you feel the indescribable feelings of self-worth and love. This is your healing power.

This increase in internal energy creates a more coherent and powerful field of energy within and all around us. This energy is something we have always had access to, and it is familiar to us because we have raised our energy (emotion) many times before. This increase of energy creates a very familiar but indescribable feeling within our being. But now we understand more about it, and we know how to tap into it at any time during our day. As this energy of indescribable feelings that are found in the feelings of love, joy, gratitude, passion, inspiration, abundance, self-love, etc. grow and become more rhythmic, we are communicating with the universe through its language. The language of vibration and frequency. Now our vibration matches with a vibration in the field all around us, and signs start to appear. Just as the G string of one guitar causes the G string of another guitar to turn on.

Now we have personal evidence that we did something internally to create something externally, and this makes the feeling of love and awe grow even more. We are hooked. We want more. We will never stop creating because now we realize we are the creator of our external reality. We realize what power we truly have within us.

## Quick Takeaways from Meditation

1. The symbol or word meditation means to become familiar with in the Tibetan culture.

2. The whole point of meditation is to become aware of where our attention is going during our waking day.

3. By sitting our body down to meditate, we are teaching it that we are in control, not the subconscious programs that have been running the show. (This is the work.)

4. In meditation, as we catch ourselves moving away from our focus and into the habitual thinking programs, we simply bring our attention back to the meditative focus we have chosen.

5. Every time we bring our attention back to the present moment is a victory.

6. There is no such thing as a bad meditation.

7. To meditate effectively, we must eliminate all distractions.

8. To get past our analytical mind, we must eliminate all five senses, as the analytical mind will be trying to analyze what we are sensing—use a dark room or face mask, comfortable chair, no noise, comfortable room/air temperature, soft meditative music, no food cooking or smells that will stimulate the sense of smell.

9. This allows us to enter the subconscious or Alpha brainwave state.

10. Here is the present moment, and in the present moment, all potentials exist. This is the dream state.

11. The present moment is the fifth dimension. There is no-time, no-body, no-one, no-thing, no-where. It is a vacuum of nothingness that is everything.

12. As we experience greater degrees of the elevated feelings of our future we have created, we get closer to singularity.

13. Singularity is the oneness, wholeness and the zero-point energy that is bringing all the three-dimensional world into our reality. It is just pure blackness.

14. Here in the present moment, we already have everything, so our future we have created from thought alone already exists here.

15. In meditation, we learn to feel the feelings this future will bring us as if it already happened.

16. This practice allows us to feel this feeling throughout our waking day. By feeling this during our waking day, we are no longer giving our attention to our old limiting beliefs of unworthiness, guilt, fear, doubt, etc.

17. This feeling is sending a chemical, hormonal and biological signature to the cells of our body, which is preparing our body to experience this manifestation in the third dimension.

18. Both while meditating and when we remember this feeling throughout our day, we are literally, healing, regenerating, and renewing our body and brain. This gives us clarity, energy, increased focus and greatness.

# Section Three:
# Posture

How we hold our body in space clearly demonstrates our mood. Our posture is our body's way of showing whether we are in a state of love or in a state of fear. When we are standing tall, feeling light with a spring in our step, the hormones of love, joy, peace, gratitude and abundance are flowing through our body. Likewise, when we are in these elevated states of energy, we are able to clearly measure our body's light emittance and see that it is stronger and more coherent both in and around our physical body. We will look at these measurements later in this section. Conversely, when we are stooped, dense, worried, scared, regretful, beaten, etc., the hormones of stress are flowing through our body. Our body's tissues hold on to who we are being as the new science of psychoneuroimmunology shows us and our energy field weakens and shrinks. When this stressed-out state becomes chronic, the cells are being fed the hormones of cortisol and adrenaline in a disproportionate ratio leading to tissue breakdown, pain and disease.

Think of the greatest people of our world and how they held their stature. Did you ever see Martin Luther King Jr. standing with poor posture? No way. He was the picture of greatness, standing tall, his shoulders like pillars on the side of his proud body. He embodied the truth, and his body language spoke a thousand words.

Imagine the posture of yourself after you have just received 10 million dollars. I imagine you would feel light, energetic, vibrant and tall. You would feel free. Your heart and chest would be open as you would be feeling a lot of energy in this area. The heart would blossom like certain flowers blossom when the sunshine hits them. Your spinal muscles would become more balanced and coherently defying gravity. Your leg muscles would be stable and firm, allowing your calf and ankle muscles to bound you along as if you were walking with the most technologically advanced springs. Through every step, the energy from the earth would vibrate through each step you take into every cell of your body seamlessly. You would be more energy and less matter, and your body's posture would portray this as if the earth had less gravitational pull holding you down.

In this section, we will go deep into our body's posture. We will go through each spinal level and explain the muscle balance needed for optimal health. We will start with the root or the sacrum and work our way up to the brain spinal level by level. Even above our head to our energetic aura that has been depicted as the halo in many ancient portraits. We will discuss the energy of the spine and the importance of the proper flow of cerebral spinal fluid. As we are learning about the spinal posture, we will learn about its importance to the function of the rest of the joints of our body. In the lower extremities, we will learn the correlation from our lumbar posture to our hips, knees, and ankles. And in the upper extremities, we will learn the correlation of our thoracic and cervical spine to shoulders, elbow and hand.

I will educate you on how to take your body's pain away by consciously moving the muscles of your spine to reposition the body into a pain-free state. By doing this, we must become more aware of our body. We will learn to go within and pay attention to what our body is telling us. Pain is our body's way of giving us information, and in this section, you will finally understand what to do with that information by gaining an awareness of what your pain is telling you. Just as we learned to go within and become aware of who we are being emotionally throughout the day, we will learn to do the same physically in our posture position. Mike Wasilisin has coined the term of this awareness "positional presence." Instead of looking for the outside fix from a pill, doctor, physical therapist, chiropractor, etc., we will learn how to fix ourselves. By understanding the spine and how its posture effects every joint of the body, you will be able to take control of your pain and not let it control you.

This section will include a written description of how to engage, strengthen and balance the muscles of the spine and upper and lower extremities. In addition to this, I have created video tutorials via my website, breaking down all sections of the body. This will allow you to focus on one problematic area of your body and heal it, or on a grander scale, learn how everything in our body is connected. You can find all the video tutorials of everything from this section at casonlehman.com/wth

During our dive into the explanation of the muscles, their location and their effect on the spine, we will also go into detail about the eight energy centers of our body. These centers are what are known as the chakras. Chakra is Sanskrit and translated as *wheel*. These little but powerful energy centers of our body are just that— wheels of energy. These energy centers are a convergence point between the power of the field surrounding us (consciousness) and the physiology of our physical body. Each of these centers is a unit responsible for the production of the hormones that create health in our entire body. These energy centers control the core emotional and physical functions of our being and body. We will learn where each center is located in the body and what each center is responsible for creating. We will learn how individual centers are connected to our posture and how the awareness of both our postural muscles and these centers will improve our health through the new sciences we have learned. We will learn how if these energy centers are out of balance or congested it affects our vital life force and creates dis-ease.

Finally, I will introduce you to another very powerful healing meditation, where you will place your attention, and therefore your energy, onto each of these energy centers in your body through a meditative process. In this meditation, you will practice placing your convergent attention and energy on each of your energy centers working the energy from the base of your spine, or first energy center, into the second and so on, from the bottom up to the eighth energy center on top of your physical head. By learning to place your attention on the energy in each of the centers, you will connect and balance your hormonal centers back into health. The energy of each center magnifies, seamlessly connecting and flowing into the next. For example, as we feel the energy from our first energy center or root chakra, we will then consciously take our attention to our second energy center. The combined convergence of the energy from one and two seamlessly ascend and equal the energy of the third energy center. Then, one, two and three rises and become equivalent to the fourth. The combination of each center's collective energy causes an ascension of vigor throughout our spine and entire body.

This will allow for an even greater super charging of healing in your body. This meditation will teach you how to place your attention on these chakras in your body to send your vital life force energy to them. Based on the principles of biophysics you will be increasing the energy of the cellular health of these centers by giving them not just your attention but your gratitude for the inconceivable amounts of cellular functions they carry out millisecond by millisecond below our conscious awareness.

## Base of the Spine. Its Nerves

Just like the rest of our physical body the spine woks as one single unit. It works in wholeness. It does have a top and a bottom, but the way it works cannot be simplified or reduced into pathways of one direction and another. Although, this does help us better understand its function, its magnificence is beyond our comprehension. At any moment in time, the spine and its nerves branching into our body like a tree are picking up information from the field both outside our body and sending and receiving that information it picks up to the inside of our body. This gives us an awareness of ourselves in space, which we have termed proprioception or the sixth sense. No matter how hard we try to explain and understand these phenomena, we still cannot comprehend the speed at which proprioception happens.

For example, in every moment, our spine is picking up every sensation via the nerves of our body such as hot, cold, breeze, touch, pressures, as well as our body's position of itself in space (so that we do not fall). All while simultaneously controlling the muscle actions of every muscle of our body to orient and navigate around our three-dimensional world. It is doing all these functions from the top down, bottom up and every way in between. It is absolutely mind bending how it coordinates all of this to the brain and then back into the body for us to function on a moment-to-moment basis.

The nerves of our body are always sending and receiving signals to our brain. Whether it is the feeling of the wind on our skin, the warmth of the sun on our shoulders or the proprioception of our ankles feeling the ground as we are walking, there is a constant rhythm of communication and information running up and down our spinal cord to be processed by the brain and then back to the body repeatedly. It is a flow that is beyond our comprehension. We can better become aware of it but without fully understanding it. We do not control it for it merely occurs, just as our heart beats.

However, we can practice becoming more aware of it as we learn to sense our body.

A general theme I hope you understand in learning about the spine and body is that it is all one. There really is no beginning, middle or end. The spine and the rest of the systems of the body are in constant communication with no separation. They are a whole. It is a unit that works together in a unison of rhythms ruled by energy or vibrations, which are always communicating within us and all around us. Our movements and actions are just changing these rhythms. In this section, we will learn how to become better connected to the energy of our body by using our free will and choosing to pay attention to it.

The sacrum roots us to the earth. It is our grounding. It helps us create a firm base for our proverbial tree to blossom. When you extrapolate the nerves from the rest of the body's tissue, it resembles a tree. In the form of the lower extremities, nerves being the roots that go into the ground, our spinal cord being the trunk of the tree, and the upper extremities being the tree's branches. See the picture below for a clearer image.

## This is Your Nervous System

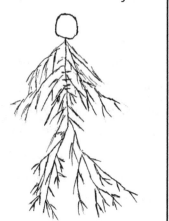

## This is a Tree's Roots

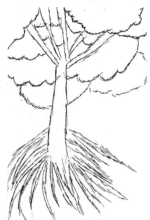

*Figure 6*

As you look at this amazing comparison sketch (figure 6) that my daughter drew, imagine that the nerves of our lower extremities are connecting us to the earth so we can feel, sense, balance and connect to the ground. The nerves and tissues of our body as well as the energetic field around our body are constantly picking up vibrations from our environment. Even if we are not physically connected to the ground, our bodies (physical and energetic) are receiving information that connects us to this physical three-dimensional world. You may liken this to the sixth sense. I am trying my absolute best to describe to you how astonishing our minds and bodies function. Throughout so much of our lives, we take this absolute wonder of what we truly are for granted. My point here is to help you remember the awe-inspiring beings that we actually are. And, no, you are not excluded!

These nerves are not only picking up vibrations from the visible earth and its structures, but they are also picking up vibrations that are invisible as you know the field is filled with information within and around us. Just think for a moment about how a human being balances on two feet. It is absolutely astounding when you think about it.

In Physical Therapy school, we learn about a term called ankle strategies, which basically is described as how the nerves of our ankle communicate to the nerves of our calves, quadriceps, pelvis, hips and then to the spinal cord, to the brain and back down again. We are taught that nerve synapses by which the nerves communicate happen via a synaptic firing between the synaptic cleft of each individual nerve up and down the nerves of our body up to the brain and back. We learn that the axon or arm-like projection of the neuron (a nerve cell) are electrically conducting this innervation by way of magnesium, calcium and other ions that are conductors of electricity all happening at a hyper-fast speed to keep us balanced by muscle contractions. This is all very interesting and essential to better understand the physiology of a human being, but there seems to be more to this amazing phenomenon of balance. We are not taught about the marvel of the speed at which all of this is occurring.

I often think about how all of this can be happening in linear time.

We also learn how the ankle strategies and the nervous system all play into balance. We learn dis-eases that affect one's balance as well as the pathophysiology of the diseases. We learn balancing exercises to help improve our proprioception by closing the eyes and standing on one foot to stimulate and improve one's balance and neuromuscular abilities. My point here is not that the aforementioned ideas are bad or wrong. I think they are great, but these ideas are not enough to explain the magnitude and brilliance of our balancing bodies in space. Just as the observer effect turns nothing into something, so, too, do our bodies turn defying gravity by standing upright into balance in a way that, to me, is a phenomenon with much more to it than ankle strategies and our current understanding of the nervous system's ability of proprioception.

As we investigate the amazing capabilities of our human body and how it is able to pick information up from the field, we start to see patterns occurring and one of the most basic but fundamental patterns of all.

The pattern we see is this:

Input >>>>> Processing >>>>> Output

Here is an example using our ability to catch ourself from a slip and fall. Our sensory *input* is picking up information in the field as we are walking—things like our brain detecting water on a marble floor directly ahead of our next step. This information is then *processed* by the spinal cord and the brain to help determine our reaction or *output*. Now our body has a motor response in the form of muscle contractions to stabilize our balance on the slippery surface. This muscle action to keep our balance is the *output*. This is all done below our conscious awareness at a quantum level to catch us from falling. To determine the speed at which the biochemical reaction of this happens is impossible.

By looking at the cross section of the spinal cord, we can better understand how our body is capable of this quantum phenomenon. The butterfly shape we see in the spinal cord is where the neurons are bundled. As we look at the image below, we see the top half of the butterfly wings, the top section is where our sensory neurons are located. These are taking in information from the invisible field of energy. This is *input*. Between the top and the bottom half of the wings are the associative neurons. These neurons are *processing* the information as it is coming in. They process and make sense of the information sensed. And finally, we have the motor neuron bundle, which is the lower section of the butterfly pattern. Here is where the *output* occurs, and in the case of our amazing balance, this is how our muscles are directed to contract and stabilize our skeleton to stay upright. We will use this pattern of input-process-output throughout this section to understand how we are constantly reading the invisible field that governs our life.

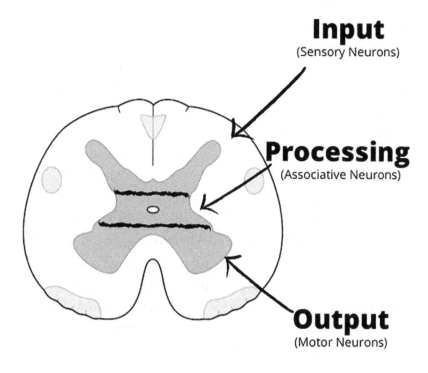

*Figure 7*

The magnificence does not end with balance. Think of all the movements the human body is able to accomplish. Dance, athletics, physical work, building, play, etc. How are we able to do all this while simultaneously our body is controlling our heart rate, body temperature, respiratory rate, the infinitesimal cellular functions, proprioception and the millions of other functions all at the same time? It is absolutely mind blowing. We are living in a body that is supernatural.

Thomas Cowan (2016) describes this mind-blowing phenomenon by starting with the explanation of the biochemistry of a nerve cell similar to what I partially described above. He points out the magnitude of chemical reactions for this nerve conductivity from neuron to neuron to finally reach its unilateral destination such as a muscle cell to fire and contract a muscle cell. Cowan makes a point that this sequence seems very clear and well worked out and that we currently adhere to a belief that because of a dysfunction in this process, there can be neurological disorders manifest in the nervous system. Diseases such as multiple sclerosis and ALS (Amyotrophic lateral sclerosis) would be two examples. Cowan points out how our current understanding is that the myelin sheaths are damaged, which causes an improper nerve conduction to the muscle tissue. The dysfunction of the myelin being the underlying pathophysiology. He continues to describe how researchers in medicine routinely try to manipulate neurotransmitters via pharmaceutical drugs. However, these interventions are affective in only some neurologically diseased patients and are only slowing the progression of the disease, not curing it. In the conventional medical world, we have settled with this pathophysiology and treatment; this is not, however, a cure. There is more to this than simply what we have settled to accept.

But Cowan asks the reader to carry out an experiment by doing the following: He asks you to have a partner to help as you close your eyes and extend both arms out in front of your body with your index finger on both hands pointing out. Then have your partner either say right or left. As soon as your partner says right or left, wiggle that index finger on the hand that your partner says. Do it three times. Now he asks you to answer this question. "How long did it take between hearing the word right or left and wiggling your index finger?" He proposes that he has done this with thousands of people and that most people say only a few seconds. But this does not take a few seconds, this happens instantaneously.

Practically, it is not possible to measure the time from the moment your partner's voice stimulates a vibration in your eardrum, which incites your brain to send a nerve impulse down the spine to the brachial plexus and from there to the intrinsic muscles in your finger, making dozens of muscles fire and contract to wiggle your finger all instantaneously. Cowan describes how current scientific explanations of this do not make sense as it would take too much time for the cause-and-effect chain reactions to take place under the old paradigm of Newtonian Physics. I agree. These phenomena happen, however, in no time at a Quantum level, which we cannot see and which we so far have not yet been able to explain scientifically.[7]

My point here is this—we are energetic beings, and we have tried to reduce our magnificence down to a scientific biochemical understanding, yet we still cannot figure it out. Because the mainstream medical narrative concentrates on only the physical, this has taken us away from our own invisible intelligence. The spiritual and energetic component of us. We are no longer listening to our gut or our heart because we have been conditioned to listen to what "they" say. Who are "they" and how did "they" become the authority that knows more than the infinite intelligence of our body? The answer is very clear. "They" have been molded by a pharmaceutical industry that profits from the masses believing a pill, a surgery or an injection (all billable) is the only thing that will "fix" your ailment. This propaganda shuns all other healing approaches as quackery by claiming it is not evidenced-based science. However, too much of the science today is funded and manipulated to reach a certain agenda's narrative.

There is nothing wrong with science. I love science, but when the science is skewed by certain agendas, then it is no longer science as there is no honesty or morality in it. The whole point of science is to demystify the unknown, viz. to bring an understanding of what we do not know. Science should be questioned and retested. And when something better is proven, it should become the new paradigm. But paradoxically, the old, outdated science seems to still be holding strong, (i.e. matter to matter) when science has clearly proven that the invisible world of electromagnetic energy has a much greater effect on matter than matter itself. I think science can bridge the gap between the worlds of the dimensions, however, when we wait for science to prove this, we are giving our innate power away to it, especially if that science is being manipulated by the dollars that funded the research.

## The Pelvic Floor

The perineal or pelvic floor muscles are the primary movers of the bottom of our pelvis. When contracted, these muscles lift our internal organs up and tighten the sphincter muscles of the vagina in women and of anus and the urethra in both men and women. These are the muscles that we use for going to the bathroom, sexual intercourse and in females giving birth.

If you were going to urinate and you needed to stop urinating mid-stream, these are the muscles you would pull up and in, stopping the flow of urine. These are the muscles involved in what we know as the Kegel exercises, which were created by a gynecologist in the 1940s by the name of Arnold Kegel. The pelvic bowl gets pulled up and inward toward the middle of the pelvis.

Practice this right now by sitting with equal pressure on both ischial tuberosity bones (the bones you sit on), your feet flat on the floor and an erect spine. Now pull the space between your tailbone (sacrum) and the pubic area of your pelvis up and in. You are pulling directly upwards toward your head. Imagine if you needed to stop your urine and activate those muscles. It may help to sit on a small rolled towel straddling it like a bike seat to feel pressure on these muscles. This will give your brain feedback with the pressure of the towel pushing into these muscles. Contract the pelvic floor muscles for five seconds, ten times. Do this as many times throughout the day as you can. The more you practice this, the more grounded and centered in your body you will become, since by doing this, you are bringing your attention and therefore your dispersed energy back to your body.

Check out my video tutorial of how to engage your pelvic floor by visiting casonlehman.com/wth

This piece of the spinal posture sets the foundation for the roots of our body to be steady, strong and stable just like the foundation of the mighty oak tree. The awareness and skill of contracting these muscles might be awkward at first, but with practice you will become more and more skilled as you will be developing a neural connection in your brain in accordance with this part of your body. This foundational muscle development is a great tool for any situation in life in which we need to ground ourselves in the midst of life's many learning obstacles brought our way. During a challenging situation in our life, remembering to pull in and squeeze the muscles of the pelvic floor can root us and help us stand firm in our self-confidence. This gives us our power back.

By practicing this muscle awareness, you are focusing your attention and therefore energy on yourself as you have learned this is essential for change. We must become more aware of where our attention is going. We have learned how to become aware of our default thoughts and emotions in Section Two, and now it is time to become aware of our body. It is time to bring our attention back to our body. Throughout our daily lives, we have our attention scattered in so many different directions it causes us to lose focus of ourself. We truly have no greater relationship than the intimate relationship with self. Unfortunately, most of us have forgotten this relationship with ourselves. And when we come home to our self, we become empowered. We see that we have choice and free will. We start to learn and know our body, and what it can do. This helps our focus and in itself becomes a form of meditation. After all, in Sanskrit, meditation means to become familiar with.

Sue Morter teaches what she calls "taking it to the body," a technique in which you squeeze these muscles of the pelvic bowl to ground yourself to the stable energies of the earth in a stressful situation of your life. I have found that this works very well when we become more aware of our body in these situations and bring our energy back to us, as opposed to letting our energy be dispersed to the person, place or thing of the perceived stress. We now are not the victim of our external environment but instead the creator of it as we learn to have better energy management. By being the masters of our own internal state by "taking it to the body," we can remove our attention from the victim state of being back into the empowered state of being. By practicing this positional presence, we become more present in our lives as we are not giving our attention to the memory of the past or trying to predict a future outcome based on our past. We bring attention to our body's posture and gain awareness. We become present in the moment. This takes our brain away from the perceived stressor and brings us back home to our body.

This is the same principle as becoming aware of what thoughts we are thinking and what kind of person we are being day in and day out. Just as we have subconscious programs of habitual thought and subsequent feeling patterns, we have subconscious postural patterns as well. As we bring our awareness to our body and correct its position in space, we start becoming conscious of our subconscious default modes both mental and physical. Both practices create the same effect of bringing us to the present moment and focusing on who we are being. This postural presence is crucial in creating our new self as well as living a pain free life.

Now that we understand the first postural checkpoint to set our unshakable foundation, we can now ascend from it.

## The Butt, Sacrum and Pelvic Tilt

The second postural check point that we will learn are the muscles of the gluteus maximus and the sacrum otherwise known as the tailbone. This is your butt (gluteus maximus). This group of muscles is one of the biggest and most vital in the human body. Many teachings tribute the gluteus maximus muscle as being the most important muscle in the body as it connects and balances the top and bottom half of our body. I have found this butt muscle to be very underutilized in many patients with ankle, knee, hip and spinal pain and dysfunction. Because of this underutilization, the coordination of voluntarily contracting this muscle is, in many, just not there. Nerves that fire together wire together. Therefore, just as we practice the feelings of gratitude, love, abundance and freedom to build and grow new neural networks in the brain to allow these higher vibrational feelings to expand, we also have to practice the contraction of our weak postural muscles to ensure their growth. The more we fire these muscles (contract), the more we wire our connection from brain to body, making a lasting connection.

The sacrum sits at the base of the spine like an upside-down triangle. It has the ability to rock forward and backward, known as nutation and counter nutation. To nutate means to nod. The tailbone can nod back and forth where the tip of the triangle will move forward (anteriorly) toward the front of the body and then backward (posteriorly) toward the back side of the body. This movement of the sacrum is important to understand as we learn to engage the gluteus and perineal muscles. Look at Figure 8 to see how the nutation of the sacrum operates.

# Sacral Movements

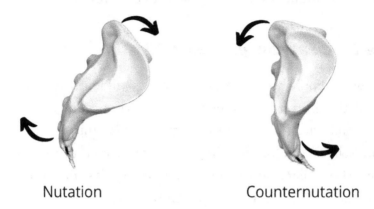

Nutation                    Counternutation

*Figure 8*

The gluteus maximus or butt muscles are essential in the balancing of our pelvic tilt. The pelvic tilt is the forward and backward hip thrust and unthrusting movement of our anatomy, which coincides with the nutation and counter nutation of our tailbone. The best way to describe this movement is the sexual thrusting of the hips used during intercourse. Figure 9 will give a better understanding of the posterior and anterior pelvic tilt.

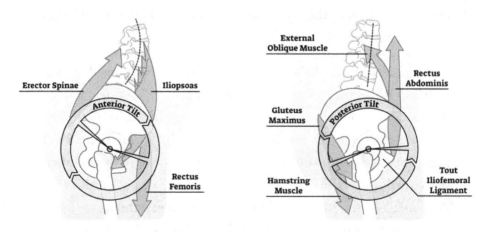

*Figure 9*

150

As we squeeze our gluteus maximus, the iliac crest of our pelvis tilts posteriorly or backwards, and at the same time the bottom of our tailbone goes forward. The iliac crest is what you set your hands on when resting your hands on your hips. The terminology used may get a little confusing, but do not get caught up in the words. Instead, feel and learn the movement using the pictures and videos found at casonlehman.com/wth to guide you. Most of us are living with the pelvis in an anterior pelvic tilt. This is when the tailbone moves backward and up, and the iliac crest rotates forward as shown in the picture above.

When we have a balanced and strong low back and hips, there is nothing wrong with the anterior tilt. It actually is a built in shock absorber, but as you can see in Figure 10, this puts a strong bend or lordosis in the lower spine (exaggerated lumbar curve), which can manifest as many joint dysfunctions, nerve impingements with pain, and muscle weakness and imbalances.

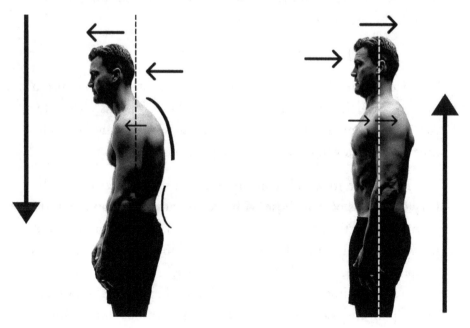

*Figure 10*

To better learn and practice this movement of the pelvic tilt, it is easiest to lie on your back on a firm surface with your knees bent and head and neck in a comfortable position. Practice squeezing your glutes and tilting the tip of the tailbone up toward the ceiling (posterior pelvic tilt combined with sacrum nutation). You can also perform this movement sitting and standing. (Sitting is a little more challenging because of the increase flexion of our hip joints.) Standing may be easier for you to solely contract your gluteus maximus. As you do this laying on your back with your knees bent, feel your lower back uncurving and straightening toward the surface you are lying on. I describe this as pressing your lower back to the floor or mat. Many times, this movement alone will take away low back pain, hip pain, radicular nerve pain, mid-back pain and sometimes even neck pain. This is setting the foundational piece of the whole spine posture where we are building the neural networks to develop coordination and awareness of this part of our body. Another great position to practice this posterior and anterior pelvic tilt is on your hands and knees. Practice all positions and do what feels best for you.

See casonlehman.com/wth for video tutorial

**Side Note-When doing this movement, if available, use a mirror to watch your body's movement. As your pelvis tilts posteriorly, your lumbar spine will open, elongate and straighten. The mirror will give you feedback to see your body's position.**

The degree to which you tilt your pelvis is something to be very conscious of. For those with severe back pain, too much tilt in either direction can result in more pain as the inflammation between the vertebrae of the spine is pushing on nerves. There is a moment in between that is our sweet spot. This point takes the pain away. Taking the pain away is the whole point. When we are in this pain-free sweet spot, the body is now primed and ready to heal, and that's what it does best. It heals.

We are responsible for giving it the right conditions to do so. These conditions we are giving it are the point of this book. Let us review what we are doing. First, we must become aware of stress and how it is running in the background, catching it in its act, and then choosing the feelings of love, joy, abundance, gratitude and a love for life we have generated from our written work. Now these emotions are turning on genes that heal, restore, regenerate and balance our body's energy and therefore chemistry. As we live in this high vibrational state of love, we now embody this with the correct and pain-free body posture and the proper food to nourish and feed our body.

## Pain is Information—Not a Bad Thing

To heal ourselves, we must understand pain. Pain is our body giving us information we must listen to. Pain is a universal nudge that we need to wake up and do something about. Pain can be a very debilitating experience because, quite frankly, it does not feel good. Oddly, however, it is very common for many of the patients I have worked with to avoid chronic pain by ignoring it. By avoiding it and ignoring it, they become blind to it. They even have a hard time describing how it feels, when they feel it, and where the pain actually is in their body because they have avoided it for so long.

Pain is information we must tap into and face. We must acknowledge our pain and respect what it is telling us. This is not information we should ignore. By listening to and facing our pain, we are growing the awareness of our physical body. We must be aware of the pain and go within to work on what or why it is informing us.

On the flip side of ignoring our pain and becoming numb to it, I have noticed in my practice that many patients do the opposite and feed off pain, pushing it to its limits. They crave pain and work through it. Both create an imbalance in the body, leading to an undeniable pain they can no longer live with. Now, because of conditioning, we "think" some expert with a special degree is going to magically fix us. In doing so, we ignore our intuitive and innate capacity that we have within to heal ourselves.

Pain is necessary in life because without pain there is no growth. This is not a physical growth I am talking about, although it can be, since muscles grow after they reach a certain point of exhaustion. I am talking about personal, energetic and spiritual growth. Opportunity exists within pain to learn who we truly are.

Deeper rooted chronic pain occurs when we are unaware of either of the two previous examples of pain. This can be broken down into craving and avoidance. In the first example, the imbalance occurs because of the avoidance. In avoidance, we tend to compensate our body to avoid the pain, causing further biomechanical imbalances. We avoid activities that we love because of the pain. We avoid using the muscles that cause the pain, and in turn, these muscles weaken, further causing a trickle-down effect of more dysfunction. Conversely, in craving, let us say we have made up our mind to walk a certain number of steps every day, but in doing so we experience and push through great knee pain. Through craving, we believe we need to push through and get stronger while unknowingly we are creating further imbalance and accelerating wear and tear.

Most of us have learned through societal conditioning (what "they" say) to look outside ourselves to "fix" our pain. Whether it is a pain pill, pain cream, doctor, chiropractor or physical therapist assistant, we tend to believe something out there is going to fix us. But this keeps us spinning round and round looking for answers when the surgery does not fix our chronic low-back pain. Or when the pill we are taking gives us one of the page-long lists of side effects. There comes a point when we realize this outside-in approach is not working, and we start to look within and say to ourselves, "What am I doing? You call this living? I have had enough." At this point, either consciously or subconsciously, we realize we must be responsible for our own health.

When we develop the knowledge, technique and skill to relieve and fix our pain at its root, we, in turn, take our power back. This is the power that is keeping our heart beating, digesting our food and allowing stem cells to activate the growth of new cells every second of every day. When we learn to harness this energy, we unleash our true potential and greatness through raising our awareness, consciousness and energy.

Now, because we have sat with ourselves in the fire and faced who we actually have been being, we can see some incongruences of avoidance and craving come up. Maybe, subconsciously, we are scared of pain, and the ego finds it easier to just ignore it. Maybe, subconsciously, we feel we are not good enough, and we need to exercise through the pain to justify our worth and prove ourselves. Who knows? The point is we have to face the pain and that, often times, is more than mere physical pain. But when we can admit, surrender and let go of who we have been, realizing we are loved, we are liberating the stuck energy causing the problems in the first place. The ego's tricks are going to make it very scary, but remember, on the other side of the fear is the freedom of a pain-free life.

## All Connected

When we engage our glutes and pull the perineum up and in, there is a chain reaction that occurs down the legs and into the feet and toes. As our gluteus maximus activates, it pulls and rotates our femur externally or outward (see Figure 11 supination). When the femur rotates externally it then causes the knee joint to be in a more unpacked and open position, turning the knees slightly in a more bowed position. All joints benefit from this. Everything from the low back, pelvis, sacrum, hip joints, knee joints, all ankle joints and all cellular tissue in between. It is all about balance in the body, and this glut activation is where it all starts. This covers a lot of potential dysfunction in the body.

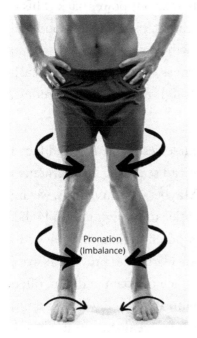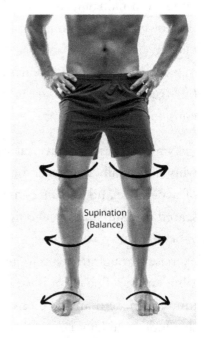

*Figure 11*

To give you an idea of how important and over reaching the lower spine and hip posture is, here is a list of some orthopedic dysfunctions and diseases that can be prevented, healed and reversed from a proper balanced posture. Low-back pain, nerve pain, sciatica, muscle cramping, muscle ache, muscle burn, any lower extremity numbness or tingling, neuropathy, hip pain, greater trochanteric bursitis, Iliotibial (IT) band pain, runner's knee, knee pain, knee arthritis, hip arthritis, low-back arthritis, degenerative disc disease, spondylolisthesis, spondylosis, scoliosis, patellar tendonitis, patellofemoral pain, chondromalacia, patella subluxation, knee pain, chronic knee pain, meniscus tear, pain from meniscus tear, bone on bone knee pain, Achilles tendonitis, non-full thickness Achilles tear, Achilles pain, plantar fasciitis, foot pain, ankle pain, ankle sprain, chronic ankle sprain, big-toe pain, toe pain, bunions, pain from bunion, stress fracture in foot, fracture in foot or ankle, heel pain, etc.

The list could go on and on, but the diagnosis is not the point. The point I am making here is that many pains and dysfunctions arise from improper posture (muscle and tissue balance/health) of the lower extremity. It really does not matter what the diagnosis is or pin pointing in which specific tissue the pain occurs. What matters is being aware of the pain and what it is telling us. With this awareness, you can take the pain away. By doing this, you further prevent the pain from coming back. This is my purpose in teaching you the knowledge of a balanced posture. When you find and fix the imbalance within yourself, you are taking your innate healing power back. And with practice, attention and persistence you can heal yourself. Or I should say the intelligence of the body will heal you. We actually do not have to do any of the healing. Our job is to create the environment (emotional balance/postural balance/muscle balance) for the body to work its magic.

As the pelvis becomes more balanced and neutral, the length tension relationship between the gluteus maximus and the hip flexors (which correlate to the back and the front of the pelvis) create an opposite reaction of the anterior pelvic tilt picture in Figure 9 above. When in proper balance, the femur rotates externally and frees the knee joint from its collapsing tension (knock-kneed) and allows the arch of the ankle to spring up and unload the over pronation or collapse of the foot as seen in Figure 11 supination image. The image in Figure 12 below will further help you understand what an overloaded anterior pelvic tilt posture of the low back and pelvis can do to the overall health of the lower extremity's joints. You can see how an imbalanced pelvis can manifest in the many orthopedic functions previously listed by causing a chain reaction all the way down the leg. This works both from the spine to the feet and the feet to the spine.

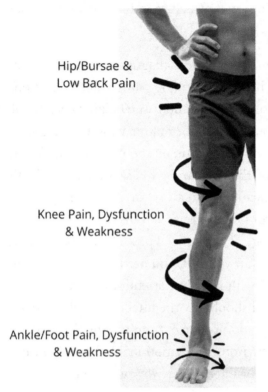

Hip/Bursae & Low Back Pain

Knee Pain, Dysfunction & Weakness

Ankle/Foot Pain, Dysfunction & Weakness

## Common Postural Imbalances

*Figure 12*

The body is one unit, not separate compartments. As you learn this, you will have a better understanding of how to prevent and take pain away when it arises. This is because of the chain of kinematics that pelvis posture down influences and vice versa. As the foot hits the ground, the muscles and joints of the lower extremity perform in a different way than when the body is not bearing weight or the foot is not touching the ground. This all gets very complicated kinesthetically, and in school, we have meticulously learned these details, but the details do not matter. What matters is your awareness of your body, how it feels and its position or posture in space. Again, if you are taking the pain away by becoming posturally aware of your body's position, that is all that matters. Pain is gone, and it feels good. As you become more familiar with your body, its muscles and how those muscles are shaping your body in space, then you have the power to do whatever is needed at any time to prevent or take pain away.

For example, you may be experiencing chronic knee pain for which you have tried many things such as knee braces, cortisone injections, physical therapy, but the pain always seems to come back. Understandably, we hone in on the knee because that is the painful joint, but there is always more to the knee pain than just the knee joint alone. In looking at Figure 12, we can see that if we do not fix the excessive internal rotation of the femur, which is done by properly engaging our gluteus maximus, then we are going to be left with knee pain. This pain can manifest anywhere in the knee (again the specific diagnosis from the MRI is not the end all be all), so we have to unload the knee from taking an improper load. Additionally, we may need to address the knee pain from the bottom up. Let us say we have an ankle that is hyper pronating (look at image 12 at the ankle). Now we have improper forces coming from our ankle up through the tibia and fibula (shin bones), driving compression into the knee joint. This imbalance can come in a wide variety of ways, but in order to create a forever fix, we must understand our entire body's posture as a whole.

When this becomes a consistent practice, the joints of the spine, pelvis, hip, knee, ankle and foot are open, youthful and spring loaded. This allows a better flow of energy from the spine to the tissues. It allows a better flow of blood. It allows a better flow of lymph fluid (which out numbers blood 10 to 1). It allows a better flow of interstitial fluid of the muscles and skin. It allows better flow of joint synovial fluid, which carries healing nutrients into the joint and extracts toxins from the joints to be funneled into the interstitial, lymph and blood to be excreted by urinating or sweating. Flow is the key, and you can see that overall flow of the body is in much better coherence. When the massive groups of cells are working in better coherence, the body becomes more rhythmic. Remember the college marching band synchronizing their cadence to create more energy? The exact same thing happens in the cells, tissues and organs of our body as the flow comes back on line.

Coherence and rhythm are health, and incoherence and disorder are the bases of disease. We are now like a free-flowing river without any manmade dams restricting the flow of water. This free flow creates more energy throughout our system, just as an untouched river carries and gains momentum. Think of how a damn affects the flow of a river. It stops the water, causing pressure to build up behind the damn. This is equivalent to an imbalanced posture. The forces taken up by the joints because of the imbalanced posture become pressurized and are like a damn blocking the normal flow of the body's rhythm.

Interstitial fluid is fluid that lives in the spaces around the cell. Its flow is essential to the cell's health. Remember cells combine their energy and production to make a tissue, tissues multiply into an organ, organs group together to make a system and systems working as one make a whole human being. As new interstitial fluid is made, it replaces the old toxic waste fluid and this old fluid is what enters the lymphatic system to be flushed out of the body. The flushing of waste is extremely important to our health as is the ability to make new fluids. When energy is low, we are not doing well either.

When our body is balanced through proper postural alignment, we are less compressed and more elongated. Our muscles, bones, joints and even organs have more alignment. This makes for a better length tension relationship in all tissues of the body. The muscles are not being kept in tension and therefore hoarding energy when they are balanced, and this creates better flow throughout their tissue. Just as the undammed river flows unobstructed, so does our body's energy and fluid. Joint spaces are open, springy and youthful. Now the cells of all these tissues are coherently operating at maximum potential with the proper spacing to do so.

Water is a conductor of electricity, and our body is made up of 70% water. This interstitial fluid is a big majority of it. Imagine that if it is working optimally, our energetic current throughout our body, which is constantly flowing, will increase. As the current increases, our light or energy is magnified.

All our trillions of cells are filled with 70% or more water in their cytoplasm. This structured water holds together like Jell-O®. Cells communicate with each other via the vibrations of this water. When the cells of the tissues are in better alignment, they can excrete their waste products into the interstitial fluid properly. When they are not filled with toxins and waste, they function optimally. As we raise our emotional energy into the states of loving life and gratitude to be alive and we hold our posture in alignment with that energy, our cells are humming at a much more orderly and coherent pace, meaning all their functions are too. The better the cell functions, the better the tissues function, the better the organs function and the better our entire body functions. This circles back to give us more energy to hold our posture in its proper place. Now we are our own generator of greatness, health and love in our life. This magic comes from within, and we realize we are the creators of it.

When we are chronically living in stress (fear), many important systems, organs, tissues and cells are constricted and incoherent. Our posture is stooped, contracted and imbalanced. We have stuck energy in our tissues like the water behind a dammed river. The flow is not equal and coherent, and pain and disease manifest. As we become aware of our state of being in connection with our posture, we have the free will to choose what to do. This is freedom. Will we let the circumstances of our life control us? Or will we choose to be greater by not allowing ourselves to fall victim to what we cannot control? In other words, will we be a victim or be the creator of our destiny?

When we choose to take our power back and lift our body up by engaging the postural muscles, we open our body's tissues. We create flow as the body must react biochemically to feed the muscles and related fluids to the tissues. We unload our joints and defy gravity by creating a more balanced space in them. We change our mind and realize we do not have to be a victim of the things we cannot control. We realize we have the power to control our inner state of being no matter what has happened in our outer environment. Now we are the masters of our body and feel gratitude for that simple yet amazing fact. Our energy raises and our tissues and cells function in a more coherent and healthy way. We are vibrating at a higher frequency. We feel better. We continue to milk this feeling more and more. Now our health starts to spread throughout our body. Now we know we can choose to do this any second, any day, at any time for the rest of our lives. As we practice day after day, no matter the outer circumstance, we turn up our awareness one small notch at a time and generate momentum for the cells of our body to heal us, this becomes our new normal, and we love how wonderful it makes us feel.

## First Energy Center. Creation

The Energy center or chakra associated with the perineum, pelvic and sacral region of our body is the first of the eight energy centers we will learn about. The first chakra is called the root chakra for good reason as it grounds our physical body to the earth. Many of the nerves that innervate the lower extremities of our body come from this region, and these very nerves are what feel and connect to the earth. Grounding is a technique in which our physical body connects with the earth through the earth's electromagnetic field. As we learn to engage the muscles of the first energy center, we will be increasing our awareness of the groundedness in our body. The practice of taking it to the body and pulling the perineum up and in is the exact engagement and awareness we will practice to become more and more aware of this energy center.

Before we move on to each of the Energy Centers of the body, otherwise known as the Chakras, I want to give a brief description of these wheels of energy to help you better build a ideal in your mind and create the healing and health of your body. Remember that our bodies are both energy and matter. The better the coherence, rhythm and flow of energy in and around our bodies, the better our cells operate (matter). Where we place our mental focus is where we place our energy, and as we learned from the observer effect, our attention is extremely powerful information the field is constantly using to create the invisible world of the quantum into matter. Because we are living in a body made of matter and energy, this means we have the power to affect the cells of it with our own consciousness. The more we become aware of the matter (tissue of our body), the more energy it is receiving from the governing field around it. This is the infinite power keeping our heart beating, digesting our food, creating new proteins for the structure and function of our body and an infinitesimal number of other actions simultaneously every second of the day in every single cell of our body. When we connect the tissues of our body to this infinite intelligence creating us, we are merging the order of the wave function into more coherent matter.

Each of these energy centers we will learn about have specific hormone producing tissues containing a package of nerves within them that carry their very own electromagnetic field. This field is measurable. This energy each center emits creates its own frequency, which as we go from the base of the spine up increases into a faster frequency (see Figure 13). Each energy center also has its own musical note and color equal to the frequency it emits. Color and sound are a vibration, and each have their own unique frequency or vibration. For example, the root chakra emits a lower frequency energy from its tissue, and therefore, it has a vibrational match with red as well as a vibrational match with the musical note C. In other words, when we measure the frequency of the color red and the musical note C, they match. This very same vibration also happens to match with the first energy center in our body. Furthermore, the second energy center is equal to orange and the musical note of D. This vibrational match of color, musical note, and energy center works its way up through all the seven centers within our body.

In figure 14, you will see the energy centers or chakras and their correlation to colors and musical notes. This will also give you a better understanding of where each energy center is in your body. Keep in mind this is information in the field all around us and within us at all times. This is consciousness, and we are all individual units of consciousness who are all a part of the ONE whole, known as the field.

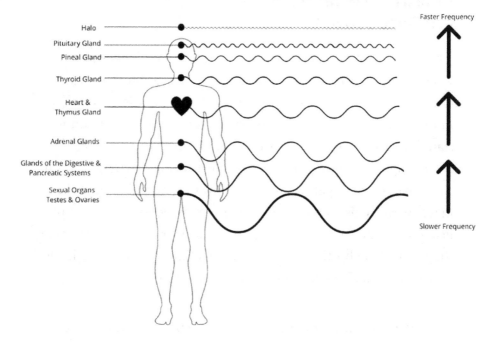

*Figure 13*

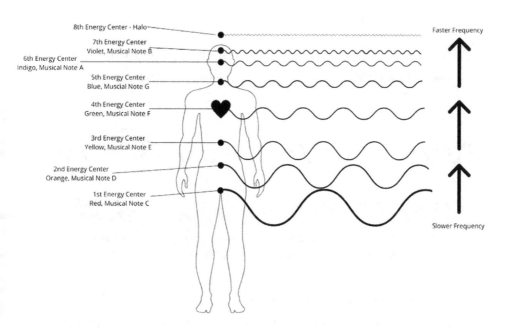

*Figure 14*

## Constructive Interference and Destructive Interference

This is what we have also heard described as good vibes and bad vibes. We are constantly giving and receiving energy, and the energy centers are the hub of much of this bundled energy, so in order to harness this energy we need to gain a better understanding of good vibes and bad vibes. Or another way to say this is the amplification of energy and the extinction of energy. When two waves come together in synchrony, they combine to make a bigger wave. This is constructive interference, good vibes or amplification. When two waves that are not in synchrony come together, they cancel each other out and dissolve into a flat line. This is destructive interference, bad vibes or extinction.

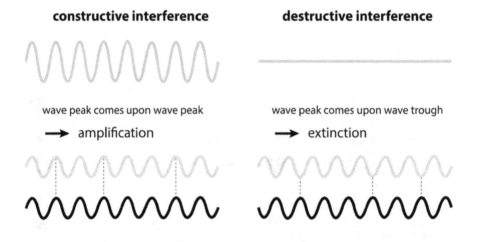

**constructive interference**      **destructive interference**

wave peak comes upon wave peak      wave peak comes upon wave trough

→ amplification      → extinction

*Figure 15 – In the amplification process of constructive interference, when two waves meet in rhythm they grow in amplitude. In the extinction process of destructive interference, when two waves connect out of phase they cancel each other out, decreasing the amplitude and therefore the energy.*

Imagine the last time you entered a room with good vibes. You can feel that energy. The feeling in you magnifies as you feel the energy of the others in the room, resulting in the total energy in the room to grow. The space is filled with constructive interference, which the coherent energy magnifies. Now imagine walking into a room where there has just been an argument between two or more people. This is a different energy you feel. These are bad vibes. The energy has been sucked out of the space of the room or is flat-lined. It is almost tangible, but very hard to describe with words.

This becomes a very important piece of knowledge to understand as we place our attention on the individual energy centers of our body. As we practice, we will begin to create constructive interference in each of these centers, creating more amplitude of energy as we work our way up the body. Starting from the first energy center, we will harness its powerful life-creating energy and coherently move it up the body through all the energy centers upgrading our body's tissues to their highest potential.

## Connections

The first energy center of the body is associated with endocrine glands of the testes in men and ovaries in women. Our first energy center has so much energy that it creates a human baby. Take a moment to think about the magnificent infinite intelligence behind this. A single-celled sperm and a single-celled ovarian egg have packed into their DNA the absolute perfect genetic intelligence to multiply enough times to make a 15-trillion celled human being. This is absolutely astonishing. The developing of this new human all happens magically below our conscious control. This means you have enough potential energy in your first center to create a human life. This energy is there for you to create with at all times. This creative energy can be harnessed and used to create the life of your dreams. All that is required is that you learn to place your energy on this area and love it for how much it does for you without you having to physically do a thing. As we become aware of this energy and we feel it more and more, we are able to connect it to our second energy center, where we repeat the same awareness process in each energy center all the way up the body to the crown of our head.

The first center is associated with the Inferior Mesenteric Plexus which are the nerve plexuses coming from the spine around the spinal nerve root level of L3 and L4. This nerve root travels to the testes and ovaries to give them their energetic flow from the spinal cord. The glands of the testes are a vital source of life-sustaining testosterone and in the ovaries the life-sustaining hormone estrogen and progesterone. When the cells of these tissues are in balance, we are full of energy, we feel at home in our own body, and we are confident in who we are. When these hormones and the tissues of the ovaries or testes are out of balance, we are over or under sexual, insecure and tend to resist change. In disharmony of the first center, we just do not feel settled and content.

Think of all the medical dysfunction associated with testosterone deficiencies in men or estrogen issues in women. We hear these issues advertised by pharmaceutical companies through our media daily. When these organs are not functionally optimally, our body is out of balance. By simply focusing our awareness on our first center, we are helping our cells regain their vitality and naturally create a balance of these hormones in the body.

As we practice contracting the muscles of our pelvic floor, we are setting the foundation of the ascension of energy through our spine and body. When doing this we are bringing our attention back to our body in a very stabilizing and foundational way. And by placing our attention on this area of our body, we are giving these cells, tissues and organs more energy. Remember energy is the primary contributing factor to our cells' health. The cells of our body do everything for us. They are constantly working for our good. They are the epitome of selfless. Our cells are the greatest team players. So, as we learn to contract these muscles and place our attention on our first center, we must learn to be grateful for all they do without hesitation for our health. By sending the emotion of love and thankfulness to this area of our body, we are creating a more harmonic energy rhythm in the tissue. When there is a more coherent flow of energy, the cells function in their innate and pre-dysfunctional way. We are thus creating constructive interference or good vibes in this center. As this happens, the cells of this center balance the hormone production to a homeostatic level, and our system as a whole gains the overall health benefit.

As we sharpen our skills of the awareness and contraction of these muscles, we will notice that in doing so we can stabilize our anxieties, frustrations and fears as they arise throughout our daily lives. Similar to a housing structure having a solid foundation or footer, we too, can set our foundation by contracting and becoming aware of this part of our body and spine. The lower vibrational feelings of anger, worry, guilt, fear, frustration, anxiety, etc. are very unstable and draining. However, as we become more aware of these thoughts and feelings throughout our day and squeeze these muscles in response to them, we become more stable and bring our attention back to the body. This practice takes our attention off the outer environment and the potential "what ifs" these emotions create and brings us back home. Our body is our home, and that is where all our power lives.

We now start to feel a great energy develop and grow at the base of our core. It feels fantastic, and it feels really familiar. This familiar feeling is the foundation of our true self. This is the base and stable footer for us to realize our true power. No more energy scattered and dispersed and utilized on judging someone, hating someone else, worrying about finances and even worrying if I locked the front door. No way! We now are aware of these little tricks our ego tries to play to keep us in the fear state. We now catch it, and we bring our vital life force energy, via our attention, back to our body as we squeeze and breathe into our first energy center.

## Lumbar and Lower Thoracic Spine

Traveling up the spinal column just north of the sacrum, we come to the lumbar region of the spine. This is the midpoint of our body which absorbs the total shock from both gravity pushing us down toward the earth and the earth's forces pushing back up through the body. It makes sense then that this bending and twisting midpoint of our body would be one that contributes to a massive percentage of a human being's pain sometime within their lifespan. According to the National Institute of Neurological Disorders and Stroke (NIH), it is estimated 80% of adults will experience back pain at some point in their life.

As we have learned in the previous section, if the pelvic floor and gluteus maximus muscles are imbalanced and uncoordinated, then the lumbar spine adopts a too extreme lordotic curve, causing the space in the back side of the spine, called the foramen, to become compressed. Refer to Figure 10.

As you can imagine, over a period with this exaggerated lordotic posture of the spine, the discs between each of the spinal vertebrae (bones) is going to give way. The forces are just too disproportional. The disc acts like a cushion or shock absorber, and when compromised, we now have a much greater chance of spinal dysfunction and pain. As we previously learned, this malalignment is manifest in every textbook of orthopedic and neurologic pathologies. The diagnosis is not the point. The point is how to prevent, reverse and forever fix the perceived pain caused by the malalignment. Our medical model is wonderful at diagnosis, but after the diagnosis, most are usually left guessing.

Now as we engage our gluteus maximus and pull our pelvic bowl up, we are nutating our sacrum and rotating our pelvis in a favorable direction to relieve the increased lordosis of our low back. With that foundation set, to further lock this spinal posture in, we must draw our most central abdomen muscle in toward our spine. This muscle is called the transversus abdominis. We will call it TA for short. To engage the TA muscle, we must pull our naval back toward our spine. Another way to think of this is to pull your belly in as if you we sucking in to button a tight pair of pants. As we contract these muscles, our base is finalized. The picture below shows the transverse abdominis and its attachment points to our body.

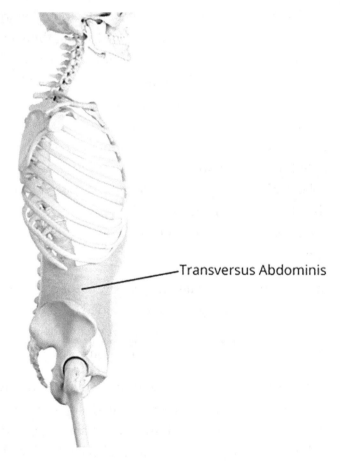

Transversus Abdominis

*Figure 16*

As you can see, the TA connects into the lumbar spine, therefore when you draw your belly in and contract the deep TA muscle, you will help straighten out the lumbar lordosis. At the same time, you will be helping the gluteus maximus tilt the pelvis posteriorly, which means the tailbone or sacrum nutates toward the front of the body. Synergistically, this is putting the base of the spine in a perfect alignment. It is now up to you to feel how much torque is needed in each different muscle group.

Before we practice, it is important to note that in some more sensitive lower-back pain patients, I have noticed the synergistic or coupled movements of both the TA and the pelvic tilt can increase the pain. This is merely because the synergistic muscle recruitment causes too much shearing on the inflamed spine. Remember, the whole point is to take the pain away or at least decrease the pain. Do not be a robot and perform the exercises without listening to your body. There is no black and white, no perfect fix. You must be your own scientist and experiment on the most pain-free position for you. Some examples of different variations could be no pelvic tilt coupled with TA contraction, less-aggressive posterior pelvic tilt coupled with TA contraction, posterior pelvic tilt coupled with pelvic-bowl contraction coupled with TA contraction. There are many more variations, however the point is for you to find the sweet spot.

Because this medical terminology is new to some of you, I know this can be very confusing, so I have a video on these variations, explaining them in the most common-sense way possible for you to visualize these positions at casonlehman.com/wth

Now, let us practice putting the lower lumbar and pelvic posture all together by gently squeezing our glutes as we pull in our pelvic floor or bowl and then draw in the transversus abdominis. This is all done synergistically and in a relieving fashion. This can be done lying on your back on a comfortable yet firm surface, sitting or standing. You can do this anywhere, really. We just have to continue the practice.

Again, remember if there is pain, our body is giving us information that something needs to be loosened or tightened. If you experience pain, do not give up and say, "See, I knew there was nothing that can fix me, I am screwed!" Trust me, there is a way. It is just going to take some practice, persistence and readjusting.

I understand this is asking a lot, especially if you have never worked with these muscles before, but remember there are video tutorials available on my website with step-by-step instructions for each spinal and energy center level. Stay with me. There is more postural adjustment that will elevate your body, mind and soul to its infinite potential.

While practicing improving our lumbar and hip posture, low-back pain can cause us to want to give up. The pain makes us irritable, angry, and frustrated, especially if it is something we have avoided for years. It's like an annoying fly we just do not want to deal with, but it keeps coming back. It is very important to understand this is your ego trying to get you to sway away from the unknown. Your pain is known, it's been there forever, and you have become accustomed to it, so oddly enough, your ego would rather stay with it because it is familiar. Facing the pain and dealing with the freedom on the other side of it is unknown and new territory. It presents itself as a terrifying place. By understanding this, you have the knowledge to give you courage to sit in the fire and face the fears avoided for so long. Keep going!

## Second Energy Center.
## Hormones and Organs

The second energy center is located just behind the naval and down about two inches deeper in the abdomen. This energy center is tied to the digestive and pancreatic hormones released into the intestines and body. The second energy center is associated with the superior mesenteric plexus of the spinal cord which originates between the first and second lumbar nerve root level. This is just above the Inferior Mesenteric Plexus where the nerves originate leading to the first energy center.

The second energy center has everything to do with proper food digestion, nutrient absorption, and elimination of wastes. This is our gut. As we become aware of this area of our body and learn to contract the muscles associated with it, we bring our energy back to it. As we learned, stress inhibits proper digestion. Digestion and the proper breakdown of food takes a back seat when we are living in the fight-or-flight state of being. Now that we are aware of this, we must bring our attention back to our second center. By simply doing this, we are turning off the stress response as we can only be in the parasympathetic nervous system or the sympathetic nervous system. We cannot be in both at the same time. By taking a moment to pause, sit down, slow our breath down and put our attention on our second center, we are turning off the stress response, letting our body know it is safe.

Remember how astonishing the tissues of the gut are, all working in a symbiotic relationship with a microbiome of organisms that are working for us? This combination is home to trillions of cells in our very own gut. All these microscopic living units have their own little energy producing, excreting and harmonizing capabilities. When this massive energy source of our body is not harmonized, we are at much greater risk for dis-ease throughout our entire body. Everything from food allergies, seasonal allergies, constipation to depression. So much stems from the health and rhythm of our gut.

Think of all the digestive diseases and food allergies so prevalent in our world today. Imagine if we started feeling our gut and sending it our gratitude for keeping us nourished and healthy. Loving our own guts for doing the moment-by-moment work of excreting and processing all the nutrients our body needs to function. By simply sending our gut this gratitude, we would be sending our vital lifeforce back to it through this focused attention. As the cells of the intestines receive their vital lifeforce energy back, they begin to work in our favor.

Peristalsis becomes more rhythmic. Peristalsis is the rhythm of the intestinal muscles contracting to push the bolus of food through the winding intestines. We begin to go to the bathroom with regularity and with much more ease. The enzymes of the gastrointestinal tract are now properly manufactured and released from the mouth, stomach, intestines, pancreas, and gallbladder cells to ensure proper food splicing, breakdown and therefore absorption. With our food broken down into the tiny nutrients our cells recognize, homeostasis of the gut tissue comes back on track. Now that we can use these digestible resources, our body receives the energy it needs to properly fuel and regenerate the rest of our tissues and all our organs.

The pH level of the intestinal cells and all its secretions become balanced, giving the gut an opportunity to start working for our good instead of constantly working to calm down the inflammation in and around it. The epithelial cells that align together like vertical building blocks mend their Velcro-like connections, healing and sealing the lining, thus keeping inflammatory agents from seeping into our blood stream. As we continue to intentionally place our focused attention to our second center, we continue to foster a balanced pH in our gut. This further decreases the systemic inflammation once allowed to leak into our body as the inflammatory agents are kept out because our gut lining has sealed. This is becoming much more manageable for the immune system to heal the cells and tissues in our gut allowing for the intestinal inflammation to be cooled as the fire is now being tended to. Inflammation is acidic in nature, and as the intestines cool off and its pH balances, so does the rest of our body.

Now that the gut is functioning properly, the large intestines function more optimally. Doing things like secreting an essential fatty acid called a short-chain fatty acid (SCFA). SCFAs are very potent anti-inflammatory agents to our entire system, created by the microbiome of the large intestines. In Section Four, we will talk about how eating grass-fed butter can help increase the SCFA production in the gut. Butyric Acid is one of the main SCFAs, and its name stems from butter as this is where it was first discovered.

## Gut Feeling. Our Second Brain

The gut is responsible for much of our intuition, so much so that it is often called our second brain. There are over 100 million neurons in the intestines in constant communication with the brain through the vagus nerve. The vagus nerve is the only cranial nerve that goes past the brainstem and into the body. This powerful communication channel connects with the majority of the abdominal organs, but most of its connections are in our intestinal tract. The vagus nerve was previously believed primarily to only send information from our brain to the body's organs. However, we now know that what our vagus nerve does is, in fact, mostly the opposite of this.

It is estimated that 80-90% of the information the vagus nerve is relaying comes from the gut to the brain. This means the gut is picking up information from our food and our environment and sending it back to the brain much more than the brain is sending information to the gut. We see here again the pattern of input-process-output. In this case, the gut is sensing very large amounts of input from the field and from the contents inside of it and then relaying it to the brain. The brain processes this information from the gut and creates a visceral or musculoskeletal output in response.

There is a fascinating bond between the microbiome of our gut and our brain. Science is just recently starting to better understand these incomprehensible wonders through the study of enteroendocrine cells (EEC). Remember how the enterocytes of the gut lining are stacked together side-by-side like blocks? Well, we now know that together within this one-cell thick gut lining are specialized enteroendocrine cells. In fact, about 10-15% of the epithelial lining of the gut is made of the enteroendocrine cell. See Figure 17 to understand how the EEC fits into the gut wall lining. Just as their name implies, these cells work as part of the endocrine system, which is responsible for the production of hormones. What is even more surprising is that the EEC are the primary producers of serotonin, which is used as a mood regulating neurotransmitter in our brain. Secondary to serotonin, the EEC also produce dopamine and other neurotransmitters.

There are afferent neurons that connect to each of the EEC throughout our entire intestinal tract and scientists have found that these neurons stick out past the epithelial lining of the gut for closer connections to the microbiome that live within us. These nerve fibers wrap around the EEC and listen to our microbiome giving the information they receive directly back to the EEC. This then is transmitted to our brain via the vagus nerve. What this means is that our brain is not only listening to our human input but also to the intelligence output of the bacteria and fungi (which are not us) living inside. These bacteria, fungi, viruses, etc. that live within our gut have been around way longer than we have, and we are clearly using the information they process for, not only, the benefit of our health but of our greater purpose here on this planet Earth. When they are imbalanced, we are imbalanced and sick. This is becoming clearer as we see the outbreak of neurologic dis-eases today. From the autistic spectrum in children to the explosion of dementia in our over 50-year-old population, this is suggesting strongly that our bacteria can determine our behavior.

The microbiome creates a wireless communication network that passes electrical energy through tissue. Like your cell phone when it loses wireless connection from the surrounding towers, we can become isolated. In this cell-phone analogy, when isolated, we do not work properly. Our calendar fails to sink up, we cannot send text messages, our calls drop. We are disconnected from the greater network. In this disconnection, chaos ensues and without seeing outside of the chaotic box, we malfunction and become irrational thanks to the stress this creates. The same thing occurs in the gut. When the microbiome are imbalanced and weak, secondary to constantly living in the state of fear, overuse of antibiotics and the SAD, it becomes isolated. The wireless communication network of these brilliant tiny organisms are cut off from our tissues. This disconnect ultimately leads to inflammation and chronic dis-ease.

As there is a disconnection of our microbiome and our own inherent cells, all the organisms, including our own cells, function very selfishly and are not working for the greater good, just for their own survival. Our microbiome, these bacteria, fungi, protozoa and viruses we have vilified as dirty and pathogenic are actually a part of the mother earth living inside us. They are much greater than what we currently comprehend, and we are just starting to learn how their powerful methodologies as a species have liter-ally allowed our existence here on planet earth to evolve. It has never been more evident than now as we have attacked them in a war-like fashion only to see our health and dis-ease decline out of control.

Through this understanding, we can better comprehend our interconnection to mother earth through these ancient microbes living within our gut. The intelligence of these organisms is in constant communication with the nervous system of our body, uploading information wirelessly from the field directly into our being.

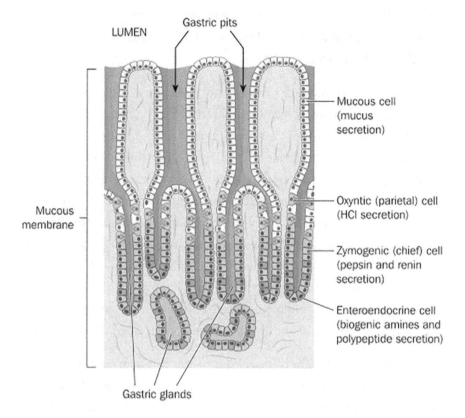

*Figure 17 – Notice the Enteroendocrine cells are the darker shaded cells scattered in abundance throughout our intestinal lining. These cells are in direct communication with our brain, sending instant messages through their respective afferent nerves, then to the Vagus nerve and finally into the brain. This shows us how our gut is very literally our second brain.*

Speaking of sensory input, our sensory nervous system can be up to 1000 times more abundant in nerve count than our motor nervous systems. What does this mean? Well, simply put it means we have all the tools we need to heal and repair, as our body is constantly sending our brain information. This is information from the field around us and from within our own cells, tissues and organs. As we begin to practice feeling or sensing our second center as well as the rest of them, then we become more in tune with our innate selves. This is our invisible, energetic body that already knows what to do. This is our gut instinct. As we practice keeping our attention on our body, our body innately uses the tools we already have from within.

I have been practicing bringing my awareness and attention to my energy centers by using the different Joe Dispenza meditations for years now, and what I have learned is that subconsciously I did not feel safe. Consequently, I always had trouble with my gut. From gluten intolerance to dairy intolerance to an anal fissure (not fun) to being nervous and constantly having diarrhea. My gut was a wreck. I always had to know where a bathroom was, and I had to have my Preparation H® wipes with me as wiping was excruciating. After I stopped eating gluten, dairy and sugar, my anal fissure calmed down and healed, but then I actually became scared of gluten and dairy. I accepted that I would never eat those two foods again for fear the inflammation in my gut would come back.

However, as I learned more and more about myself, my own healing capacity, and I did the work of the meditations, I began to realize I was living in a state of not being safe all the time. A state of fear. I realized that when it came to food, the bathroom, travel or anything out of my comfort zone, I instantly and unconsciously got sucked into the state of fear. A story in my head constantly ran. "What am I going to eat that is safe?" or "Oh no! What are the ingredients in this. It could hurt me." Simply put, I was giving my power to the food. As I was unconsciously living in the state of stress, this took the energy away from my gut that it needed to heal itself.

By placing my attention and love into my second center, gradually I started to feel safe. No aha moment or mystical experience, I just realized what I was doing. I decided to experiment with food (just a little). I ate bites of organic wheat bread or had some cheese on an omelet. Sure enough, no issues with my gut. Now to be honest, I do not eat whatever I want. I still believe food is medicine, so I am very mindful with my food choices. However, when traveling or going to eat dinner with friends and family, I catch this fear that arises and know I am greater than it. I go within and send focused attention to my gut, knowing it has the power to keep me safe.

I can now trust my body to take care of toxins coming in. In doing so, I healed and sealed the lining of my gut. Or should I say, again, that my gut and innate wisdom of my body healed itself. Fewer toxins enter my blood stream as the gut is sealed. The epithelial cells have returned to balance and rhythm manufacturing and regenerating at their peak performance. My immune system has ramped up its magnificence, catching any undigested food or toxic chemical that slips through the lining of my gut, stopping them dead in their tracks. We will learn about the energy centers associated with the immune system as we learn about the third and fourth energy centers in the next few pages. This was all done by my body. It is magic and only left for us to continue learning more about. All I had to do was sit my butt down in my meditation chair and place my energy in my energy centers, no matter how much my body wanted to get up.

With practice we learn to trust our gut. This is obviously something intrinsic to our human nature, but we have become disconnected from it thanks to the hormones of stress. By repetition of focusing our attention on our second center, we feel the familiar emotion of safety. We trust. Safety is huge in creating our health or anything we want in our life for that matter. Just think about our two autonomic nervous systems. If we do not feel safe, we are definitely in the fight-or-flight nervous system. However, when we feel safe and secure, our body starts to regenerate, assimilate, repair and heal because the energy for it to do so is available. As we practice feeling safe and relaxing into this feeling in our second center, we tell our body it is ok. We turn off the fight-or-flight nervous system we have been so accustomed to live in. We trust our innate intelligence to heal. This is largely due to the fact that we feel connected to something greater than ourselves alone. We become aware of how much fear was controlling all our decisions, and we come home to a very familiar and relieving feeling in our gut.

Food is a large part of our safety. Have you ever heard of comfort food? As we now better understand, stress (fear) can induce reaching for higher carbohydrate 'comfort foods' to satiate our need for safety. When the gut, which is constantly sending massive amounts of information to the brain, is triggered to feeling it is unsafe, anxious or worried, many times an unconscious temporary relief to calm that feeling is to eat. High carbohydrate, ultra-processed food is designed in labs by humans to be nearly irresistible to the gut-brain axis. It is as if we are being programmed to eat these major food company's foods they create in a laboratory. Hint, hint—we are. When these foods are consumed, fungi-like candida albicans overgrow in our gut microbiome. Candida feed on sugar and become overgrown in our gut. What messages do you think they are sending to the brain via the vagus nerve? FEED ME SUGAR, NOW! They are deafening and selfish.

Now imagine you can bring this feeling of safety and love to your second center. Imagine by simply bringing your awareness to this center that you create more wholeness, coherence and vitality to these trillions of cells. Imagine you can choose to be greater than the food cravings because you know at any time during the day, your own consciousness can give you this feeling of safety. Imagine having that level of awareness and self-control. You do!

We have all done this before, as we brought our attention to our body and into our second center, we experienced a wide variety of feelings that have guided us in making the right decision. Although our gut intuition is very hard to describe, it is a familiar feeling we can all tap into at any time. The gut has its own mind constantly communicating with the intelligence of the body. All we need do is tap into this area of our body and place our loving intention on it frequently and allow it to do what it does naturally.

## The Core Brace

Working our way up the spine, we now must learn to engage our outer abdominal muscle to brace down our ribcage and mid-thoracic spine. Using your fingertips, grab under your lower ribs just below your chest and pull your fingers in, gently wrapping them under the rib cage. As we engage these muscles and have proper posture, we are unable to slip our finger tips under the ribs because the abdominal muscles are aligned and firm. This is a very underutilized movement in many of my patients posture and is foreign to most people. This movement alone can alleviate many pains along the whole spine, ribcage, chest, shoulder blades and shoulder joint.

Tip—If you are struggling with this muscle contraction, one technique that might help is to take a big breath in and then exhale slow and long, and continue exhaling past the point of where you would normally stop your exhale. In doing this elongated exhale, you will contract your abdomen to help you continue pushing your breath out. This is the muscle engagement we are looking for.

Another important note when contracting the core brace is not to allow the shoulder and scapula to roll forward as the core braces and contracts. You will become better aware of this in the next section of the spine when we learn about the position of the shoulders and shoulder blades.

To see a video demonstration of this core brace engagement, go to casonlehman.com/wth

## Third Energy Center. Power of Life

This energy center is located in the pit of the gut a couple inches below the sternum. The Solar Plexus. This is the center associated with control, personal power, self-empowerment, self-esteem and the power to transform. When we are balanced in this center, we are sure of ourselves in a positive leadership kind of way. Not an arrogant gimme, gimme take, take kind of way. We are an example of greatness.

When this center is imbalanced, it can manifest as lacking self-confidence and sense of self. We say yes when we really want to say no, and we do not believe we are good enough to take on the challenge. As this center is out of balance at the opposite end of the spectrum, it can surface as greed, not letting go of control, force and power trip.

We often think of the third energy center as a bad or greedy center and shy away from it. If it is imbalanced and over dominant, it certainly can be. However, this energy center in most is under-utilized as many of us are subconsciously unworthy to receive the abundance of the universe. I certainly was. I did not realize I did not feel worthy to receive good things in my life. All my self-confidence came in the form of hoping and wishing if I just worked harder, somebody would give me something or someone would notice me. I forgot how to tap into what the universe is always giving. I thought I had to force it to happen or try harder and get what I was searching for out of material things.

I realized, however, to receive this constant gift of love the Divine is always offering, you must let go of your control and force. As I practiced my daily meditations, I realized I did not know how to feel loved, yet that is all I really wanted. I wanted to be loved and accepted by my mother and father. Because of that, in some unknown way, the subconscious program I created tried to gain approval by working really hard to impress people. As well as trying to control, manipulate and try somehow to get people to think I was successful, semi-famous and popular. Subconsciously, I just wanted to be loved.

Through meditation, I realized my inner child wanted love. I, number one, could love myself and give myself everything I always longed to have through self-love, compassion and forgiveness of myself. Second, I realized that God, the universe, the divine, whatever you call *it*, loved me no matter what. I then started to actually feel that, and I started letting it love me. This created elevated feelings of worthiness and connectiveness. I no longer felt as if I had to prove anything. I knew I already had all I was searching for. I too, like everyone else, am enough and can receive the bounty of abundance from the Universe.

Let me give you an example. Because all the vital life force from my first two energy centers were so out of balance, the proper balanced flow of energy from one and two to the third center was wobbly. This would lead to me grasping and holding on to old habitual, learned behaviors like comparing myself to others. As I caught myself doing this, I realized I either thought I was better than them (overactive third center) and looked down upon them. Or not as good as them (underactive third center) as I wanted something they had, like fame, sponsorship, an amazing house, a Tesla, or the ability and freedom to do whatever they wanted.

This then led to me going down the rabbit hole of millions of possible thoughts and actions. Maybe because I did not feel good enough later that day at home, I would assert my power as a father and husband taking my anger and inadequacy out on my daughter or wife. Or maybe I did not feel safe, therefore not good enough or unworthy, so I needed to create a fix by eating a box of munchkins from Dunkin Donuts. Infinite amounts of possible actions could have come from me living in this subconscious program, but that is not the point. The point is that when we become aware of these habits and how the energy centers correlate to them, we can go to the center and give it our attention. This allows us to heal and reassemble. Not to mention, it brings us back into the present moment as we bring our attention back to our body and off the environment we are allowing to anger or scare us.

The adrenal glands are directly associated with the third energy center and are responsible for the secretion of the hormones, adrenaline and cortisol. When cortisol and adrenaline are in check and balanced, they are powerful tools for our confidence. They give us energy to tackle challenges we fear. They empower us to be greater than our old habits we know do not serve us well. When the adrenal glands are out of balance, they are constantly pumping adrenaline and cortisol into our blood stream and are one of the main driving forces of cellular disfunction, tissue breakdown, pain and disease.

Americans today are living by the hormones of stress 70% of our day. As we live in this chronic state of stress, cortisol and adrenaline become wildly mismanaged in the cells of our body. Adrenal fatigue and many other hormone diseases are connected to the overly stressed lifestyle most of us are living. As we practice becoming aware of our posture and gain the knowledge and understanding of how the postural pieces of our body are directly linked to the hormonal centers of our chakra system, we rejuvenate the function of these wheels of energy in our body. As the first two centers awaken and begin to work in our favor, their coherent energy flows seamlessly into the third energy center. It is not just a bottom-up phenomenon—it can work in any order. The secret is that we first gain the knowledge of the healing power each of these centers have. Then we learn to focus our attention on them both in the area of our body where each energy center lives and in the space around them. This awareness combined with the practice of postural training of our muscles directly correlated with them catapults our energy and therefore healing throughout our entire body.

It was not until I started practicing paying attention to my third energy center that I began to realize how much control I thought I needed to have in my daily life. This was below my awareness because control was running on autopilot. I thought I was laid back. One day it hit me as I was driving to work. I realized I wanted to control the other cars on the road. Here's how it reconciled in my mind.

As I was driving to work, I noticed some anger in my body. As I peeled back the layers of why I was angry, I noticed a couple of subconscious programs running. Initially, I realized one of the reasons I was angry was because the other cars were in my way because I was trying to go faster than them. Because I could not control them to move out of my way, this made me angry. It then dawned on me that if I had to give up the control of my own car and ride in the passenger seat, it would be very hard to do. I had become a control freak. In this moment, I realized I have to let go of trying to control the outcomes in my life. I practiced the thought of simply being the passenger and letting go of trying to control the road.

Furthermore, I have since realized an even deeper layer of the onion. Why did I want to control the other cars in the road? Because I was in a rush. They were in my way because I was in a rush and trying to hurry past them to my destination. Something I continue to work on to this day is to slow myself down. I often catch myself in a hurry. So why am I always having to catch the old program of being in a rush? Well, what I have realized is that it originates from living in lack. When we do not feel whole, we are living in a program that we do not have it. It could stem from not feeling like we deserve "it." Or not feeling we are good enough to receive "it" because of lack of self-love. Remember, it is our subconscious belief that we do not have this thing in our possession, so we are tricked that to get it, we should rush around faster, believing we will get to our future faster. This all comes back full circle to an overactive third center by trying to control and manipulate rushing through my life, subconsciously believing that rushing is going to bring me whatever I am searching for faster. When you realize you already have it and embody that feeling, there is no rush.

Because of the lack of awareness, I was running a program I had learned sometime earlier in life. Thanks to my meditation practice, I was able to become more aware of my default mode and catch the incongruence of my behavior. This control issue I became aware of was something I could directly connect to my third energy center being imbalanced. Because I did not feel confident in who I was, this manifested as secretly trying to control others, especially while driving. I realized I was only affecting my health by behaving this way. I simply chose to stop, and I now focus on generating love into my heart when I drive. It is a perfect time to practice feeling the love of life.

## The First Three Energy Centers

The first three energy centers are all about the material world. To put it plainly, they are desires of the first center—sex to procreate and keep our species alive. The second center—to find and eat food to stay alive and feel safe. The third center—control, ego, power, manipulate for money, manipulate for sex, manipulate for food and manipulate to stay in power. These are all materialistic and deeply rooted in our three-dimensional world. Meaning we tend to try forcing the outcomes in our lives through competition and being better than. This separates us from the truth of the unity of all life. We compare ours versus theirs and take pride when ours is perceived better. This causes further separation, as now the others are not as good as us. This also works in the opposite way, where we look at what they have as being so much better than what we have. We become envious and feel inferior and unworthy. This is one of the major downfalls of social media. Below our conscious awareness, we often are comparing ourselves to others that we see, either better than or envious of. As Carl Jung said, "Everything that irritates us about others can lead us to a better understanding of ourselves."

When we are living in stress, we focus our attention on matter. Our five senses keep us locked into this material 3D world. We feel separate from everywhere, everything and everybody. We become selfish and live by our first three centers. It becomes very challenging to believe we are greater than our physical body as stress and our ego have a powerful effect to pull us back into our habitual program that is so familiar to us. This disconnects our connection to the infinite intelligence of the field that is always in us and all around us. We stop trusting in the Divinity, and we are again illusioned back into the programs we have learned from society to force, hoard, rush, acquire, compare and compete in order to be happy.

**First Energy Center**—We obsess about sex, consuming ourselves in how attractive we are and how attractive others are, conditioned by what has been perceived to be beauty by the mainstream media. Separating ourselves by comparing how we "think," we look to what magazines, television and social media portray as accepted. We put on different masks in the way of clothing that is "in style," hair, nails, make-up and cosmetic surgery. Yet, we still are not satisfied with what we see in the mirror. The male program and the female program take over without our awareness.

**Second Energy Center**—We obsess about food and over-consume it with greed, without consideration of where it came from or its sustainability on our earth. We do not care about how the animal it came from was raised, what it ate or if it lived a happy life. We do not care which pesticides and herbicides were sprayed

189

on it, what these are doing to our bodies or our environment. We only care about how good it tastes for our own satisfaction usually coupled with how inexpensive it is. We go through panic and fear when the foods we are addicted to are not available, leaving us feeling empty without them because they are filling an emotional void.

Having enough food is essential to our safety and when we live in lack and scarcity of not having enough, we feel unsafe. Emotions like fear, insecurity, unworthiness, victimization, suffering, etc. can all come online with our attention focused on the shortage of food. We do not like to share our food because of this, and we hoard it. When this center is in balance, we feel satisfied and at peace. Think of a delicious meal you eat with family or friends where you feel extremely satisfied and joyous. You are not miserable from over eating but perfect as the company and meal were perfect. This feeling is safe and secure. You have had enough and do not need anything else.

**Third Energy Center**—When we live in chronic stress, we spend the majority of our day controlling and manipulating our circumstances to suit our ego, unaware of anyone else but ourselves. We live in a "me first" state of being. We lack compassion. We consume ourselves in activity after activity, not letting go of control of our schedule, our children's schedule or our work schedule in order to get something we perceive rushing will get us.

We believe competition is how we get things we want by being better than. We have to win everything because loosing means we are less than. So, we fight for things, illusioned that loosing is a negative thing. No one is taught to embrace loss as an important lesson. We put borders up and say our side is better than your side, furthering separation. Our team is better than yours, and we will fight to prove that. When we see things we want and do not have, we get jealous of others who have them. We become envious of others' body shapes based on the comparison to ours. We resent others after not being able to get what they have or be who they are. We get caught in a program and forget about the most important things in our life. We forget how to feel gratitude, joy, love in our heart, and this further disconnects us from the beauty of the surrounding earth.

When we are stuck in the programs of these first three centers, they become imbalanced and we see repetitive patterns of disparity in our life. We work so hard but never feel fulfilled. For example, if we are overly controlling and manipulative to achieve more materialistic things in our life, believing happiness comes from these things, we often end up with adrenal burnout and get sick as we continue to chase the next material object. This can manifest in many ways in our health or life as perceived unfortunate events or circumstances.

The first three energy centers are vibrating at a lower frequency than the others in our body. Lower frequency means more density. More density means more matter or solid in the third dimension. This is why when energy is stuck or imbalanced in the first three energy centers, we become very materialistic. We are literally becoming more matter and less energy because our body is sucking the vital life energy from the field all around us and turning it into chemistry (matter) in our body. Now we are materialist because we only believe in what we can see.

Each individual center of our body is a smaller part of a collective whole, which communicates while attuning to each of the other centers. Like an orchestra having many sections combining to make a beautiful symphony and bringing a state of bliss to our ears. When our first three energy centers are balanced, they attune as a collective and create an ascension of energy up and into our heart. We feel love again and connect to the intelligence of the universe as we escape the grip of our materialistic nature. We feel lighthearted and full of love for life just like we did when we were children and needed nothing material to enliven us. We were just happy to experience life.

Now this energy and self-empowerment has nowhere to go but into our sacred heart. Our heart is what we have been missing. It is what has always been there guiding and talking to us on our most challenging days, but we failed to listen, believing happiness would be found in our material world. The heart has all the answers. It already knows our path before we step into it. It is our connection to our destiny.

## Shoulder Girdle and Upper Thoracic Spine

We are now standing on the most solid foundation rooted in a lower body posture that is unbreakable. Now it is time to open our heart and be worthy to receive the brilliance of this life.

In today's society, we do a lot of sitting. Our heads are forward and down, our shoulders rounded and our thoracic spine stooped forward as we are sitting and staring at our iPhone and Galaxies or working at our desk stressing about the budget. Our mind is so occupied with the material world that the last thing we are thinking about is our posture, let alone our sacred heart. We are dense, compressed and tense, putting the extra weight of stress on the tissues of our body. Thanks to our energy being totally diverted to the material world, we become more matter and less energy. This causes our tissues to breakdown.

Think about it. If we are just going to breakdown and wither away to dust, then what is the point of living. I think the point of living is to love. And to love is to create and evolve. If we believe we are just going to get old, get a disease, and that disease will slowly kill us, then that is what we will get. However, if we flip that, and refuse to be a victim of what we have been told (that we breakdown and need medicine to heal us), then we take our power back.

You should know enough by now that the power within us and all around is beyond our comprehension and can create something out of nothing. So why not create your health by using what you have learned so far in this book and change the narrative to one of regeneration and healing as opposed to breakdown and disease?

If we truly want to change, we must do it in love. The force of life is within our heart, so now it is time to open our hearts and learn for ourselves just how mighty our infinite heart is. To do this, open your chest by pulling your shoulder blades back, bringing them together and stick your chest out. Take your rounded shoulders and pull them backwards. Exaggerate pulling your blades together a little to get the feel of this movement. This moment of movement in the shoulder blades is called scapular retraction. Refer to Figure 18 for scapular positioning of this coupled movement.

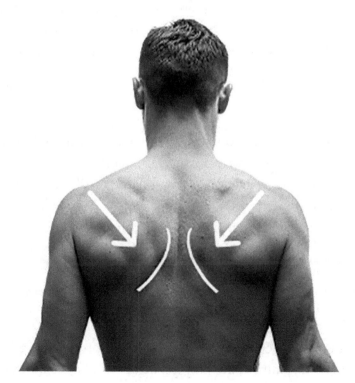

*Figure 18*

While doing this, it is important to combine the engagement of your core brace as well as being mindful of the pelvic tilt and perineum muscles. If we only pull the shoulder blades back and stick the chest out without engaging the rest of the posture below, we will create imbalance in our spine. In order not to be imbalanced, we must be mindful of all the other postural checkpoints we have learned. You do not need to contract all the postural checkpoints at once to the maximum. However, you should be able to practice this enough to the point where you can engage and be aware of them all together at once. I like to use a mirror so I can have visual feedback and go through them one-by-one, making sure I am engaging the muscles at each of the checkpoints. I find it best to start from the top down or the bottom up. From the bottom up, first we pull up our pelvic floor, then we tilt our pelvis to neutral by engaging our glutes, then we draw our belly button in by engaging the transversus abdominis, then we pull our ribcage down by using our core brace. Finally, we open our heart and pull our shoulders back by bringing our shoulder blades together.

Refer to casonlehman.com/wth for a video tutorial of all postural movements.

It might be easiest to practice the aforementioned postural ensemble laying on your back on a firm surface with your knees bent to reduce the effect of gravity on your body. This can help you learn to coordinate the movements by having the firm surface give your body feedback. Keep in mind, though, that when laying on your back, your shoulder blades will run into the surface you are lying on. You may not be able to get them exactly where you want, but that is okay. Right now, as we begin these novel movements, we are working to gain awareness and pain relief.

Remember, a coherent and balanced posture feels good. It should feel decompressing and freeing. It will be a challenge for most as this is not a familiar position to the body. The ego is going to kick in and try and get you to go back to the old default position because it is what your body knows. But the old imbalance only quickens the tissue breakdown. If we want to forever fix our chronic or acute pain, we must have postural balance with lessening or no pain.

## The Scapular Positions to Fix Pain

The scapula, or shoulder blade, moves in six different positions that are important to understand and practice in order to achieve and sustain healthy shoulders and total spinal health. The image in Figure 19 gives you a visual to gain a better understanding of these shoulder-blade movements.

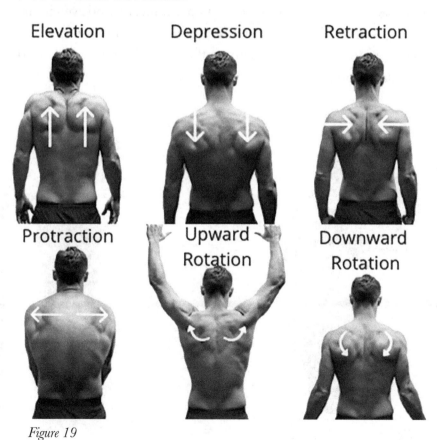

*Figure 19*

Most of us are trending toward or living in a forward head and rounded shoulder posture. This usually puts our shoulder blades into a protracted and semi-upward rotated position. This is coupled with our thoracic spine being bent too far forward (as shown in Figure 20 with the forward head and neck). As a result, our ball and socket shoulder joint, known as the glenohumeral joint, gets pulled forward, causing the rounded shoulders. Now our ball and socket shoulder joint is too far forward. This leads to many shoulder, neck, thoracic, arm and wrist pathologies. The most common I have experienced being glenohumeral (shoulder) dysfunction. This dysfunction can manifest as pain in a wide variety of areas. It can be in the front of the shoulder, back of the shoulder, in the shoulder blade itself, in the chest, referred pain down the humerus bone, in the elbow, in the upper trapezius and even in the neck. Just as the lower spine posture can cause many concomitant dysfunctions, so can an imbalanced thoracic spine and imbalanced scapular stability.

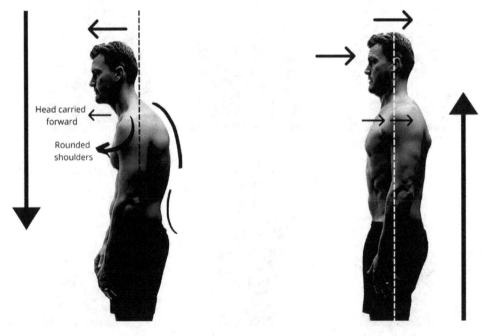

Head carried forward

Rounded shoulders

*Figure 20*

196

We can spend too much time and energy looking for the diagnosis of the tissue and lose ourselves in the medical maze. The point here is that by pulling the shoulder blades in the opposite position of the rounded shoulder and forward head, we are creating more balance and rhythm in our upper body. This would mean we need to pull our scapula into retraction and downward rotation, possibly even into scapular depression. Consequently, this is opening our heart space. Opening our chest. Look again at Figure 20 and notice the drastic difference between the forward head and rounded shoulder posture to the correct posture of me on the right.

In doing so, all the muscles of the chest are pulled and elongated back into the proper length tension relationship. The glenohumeral joint goes back into its proper place, putting the rotator cuff muscles into their respective balance. I believe this imbalance is the most common reason for rotator cuff injuries and or dysfunction. By simply opening our heart and bringing our rounded shoulders back, we are pulling our upper body back into a position for health and regeneration.

There are hundreds of details we could go into about the bicep's tendon, labrum, rotator cuff and all the other parts of the anatomy of the shoulder, but there is no point. The point is when you straighten up your thoracic spine and open your heart, you should experience less pain in whatever tissue you are having pain in.

With the posture engaged, try moving your shoulders one at a time and see how it feels. See if you experience less pain, more range of motion and easier movement by holding your shoulder blades in retraction, downward rotation and maybe some depression. I will go through in more detail all these scapular positions, glenohumeral positions and thoracic positions at casonlehman. com/wth in the shoulder pain section.

## Fourth Energy Center. The Heart

The fourth energy center sits just behind our sternum and encompasses the entire thoracic cavity. This sacred energy center is where the material world and the invisible quantum world meet. The heart is the place where the first three energy centers merge with the higher four energy centers. The connection between what we can see in our material world and what we do not see in the spiritual world. As we will discuss in more detail, our fifth, sixth, seventh and eighth centers are those of the invisible, quantum world.

For thousands of years, the heart has been known to have magical power. Many ancient cultures worshiped and celebrated the heart more than any other part of the human body, without having any of the modern-day technological sciences to confirm its magnificence. They did not need science to prove the magic of the heart, they simply lived from their heartfelt emotions. Turning back the hands of time, the magic of the heart has been shared through stories, cultural practices and epigenetics as the center of all-knowing in our body. We place our hand on our heart when we acknowledge ourselves. We hug our loved ones, connecting heart to heart. The power of love we all know and feel comes to life in the heart. The teachings of Jesus revolve around going into the heart and living from the heart. Consequently, the heart is mentioned 878 times in the Bible, and the word heart appears in 59 of the 66 books of the Bible.

Consider all the terms coined around the heart. Warm-hearted, courage, love, open heart, big heart, heart of gold, cold heart, broken heart, heart centered, eat your heart out, follow your heart, find it in your heart, to get to the heart of it, to have a heart to heart, to lose heart, to tug at your heart strings, to have a change of heart, home is where the heart is and on and on.

The heart is clearly our home. It truly is everything. It has everything we have ever wanted already in it. Every feeling of worthiness, greatness, joy, abundance, love, recognition, achievements, success. All we seek is in our heart. It has all the love we need, and it gives all the love we can give. It forgives us for our silly mistakes. It forgives others for theirs. It is where we feel grateful for our existence of life. No matter where we are in our life or what has happened in the outside world surrounding us, our heart is always there to give us courage. To encourage us to move through the fear of the unknown and see what is on the other side. We can always come back to the heart, our heart, and feel the comfort of loving compassion. It is safe, it is warm, and it is non-judgmental. It is who we truly are.

The heart has an electromagnetic field that is measurable up to nine feet away from our body. The electromagnetic field grows when we experience heartfelt emotions such as love, kindness, gratitude, abundance and joy. This field of energy can be picked up by others around us and influence their heart's field of energy (i.e. good vibes). When we focus on the heartfelt emotions of love, the heart's electromagnetic field becomes more coherent. This coherence simultaneously entrains our brainwaves into more coherence. We make clearer decisions, and we are more creative and innovative in problem solving. In fetal development, the heart forms and starts beating before the brain is even developed.

Our immune system is boosted when we are in a state of love, thanks to the thymus gland and its secretion of thymosin. The thymus gland sits directly behind the sternum and between the lungs. Thymosin is a hormone responsible for the production of T cells. T cells are a primary force in our body's defense against pathogens that can harm us and can stop them dead in their tracks. The thymus also assists in the production of B cells. B cells turn our plasma into antibodies. Antibodies seek out, find and memorize viruses, bacteria, molds and funguses that get into our system and create an internal army to eliminate them. This internal power we have is stronger than any flu shot known to man. When we place our attention and therefore energy in our heart space, we are giving this gland more energy to increase its hormone secretion and upregulate all its related cellular functions.

When we feel elevated emotions such as love, joy and gratitude, the hormone oxytocin is released from the pituitary gland in our brain. The release of this chemical through psychoneuroimmunology comes into the body and influences the release of nitrous oxide in the tissues of the heart. Nitrous oxide is known as a derived endothelial relaxing factor. This is just a big term that means this phenomenon causes the arteries in the cardium, or tissues of the heart, to open. This allows blood flow to flood into the heart. Remember that an increase of blood is an increase in energy. Our heart swells, and we feel massive amounts of energy here, allowing our heart to open and these emotions to be internalized. Now there is some serious energy in and around our entire body.

Since Rene Decartes said the heart is a mechanical pump, we have believed the heart is merely mechanical in nature and nothing more. We have settled down to accept that its only job is the pumping of the physical substances of oxygen-rich blood to our tissues and returning the deoxygenated blood back to be reoxygenated again. It is not that this task alone is not astounding. It is, but why have we stopped at this point and not looked further into the magnificence of the heart? We have bought into this belief that the heart is only mechanical in nature, and everything else seems ignored by mainstream medicine.

Thomas Cowan expands on Rudolph Steiner's theory that the heart is not a pump. Steiner, as further developed by Cowan, proposes there is no way the human heart can simply pump the blood throughout the body by alternating two movements, the contraction (systole) and the moment the heart is non-contraction (diastole). He describes the circulation as the movement of blood through the blood vessels, of which there are three types—arteries, veins and capillaries. In the capillaries, the theory of the heart simply as a pump does not make sense. These capillaries are one layer thick and a transition occurs here where nutrients and gasses are exchanged between the blood and the cells. The blood also stops, it literally stops, here to pick up waste products (toxins) from the tissues of the body. This capillary system is massive. So massive that if all our capillaries were connected end to end, they would circle the earth three times. Whoa! If they were put together side-by-side like puzzle pieces, they would take up an entire football field.

The deoxygenated blood enters the venioles from where it flows into the veins and then back to the heart. The whole point of circulation is to bring the oxygen-rich blood to all the cells and tissues of the body and then bring the deoxygenated blood back to the heart and lungs so it can be replenished again. In just this simple circulatory pathway, there are some amazing mysteries. One of which is that the blood literally comes to a halt and stops moving in the capillaries. This is essential for the life-sustaining gaseous exchange that happens between the oxygen and carbon dioxide as well as all the vital nutrients passed from the blood into the cells of the tissues. After this stopping of the blood for its exchange, the blood then starts to oscillate before it starts moving again into the venioles and then into the veins. The question that arises is, if the heart is a pump, then how does the blood stop moving for a moment and then start moving again? Would not a pump keep fluid moving at a constant flow? And if the fluid did stop moving, there would have to be another pump where the fluid has pooled to move that fluid again after it has stopped. However, there is no such pump in the capillary system of our body. This would mean then, that since the blood stops in the capillaries, there must be a force to move the blood up and back into the veins from the capillaries themselves. The heart being just a pump could not do this.

Cowan goes on to describe how the fourth phase of water is responsible for this movement of blood again after it has stopped in the capillaries. Gerald Pollack has spent many years of his life studying water and has found there is a fourth phase of it. This phase is known as structured water or the gel phase of water. We have learned that water only exists in three phases such as solid, liquid and gas. However, a fourth phase of water has a jelly-like consistency to it. This fourth phase is an intermediary state between the liquid and the solid phases. In fact, every cell in our body uses this phase to keep its cytoplasm intact. The structuring of this water in our cells is why our cells do not leak as if they were made of the liquid phase of water. Our cells are made of 70% water, and that water is in the state of the fourth phase.

The fourth phase of water has some amazing energy producing effects to it, and this is how the circulation continues from the capillaries to the veins and back to the heart. This is the moment when the blood has stopped in the capillaries to allow the nutrient and gaseous exchange as well as the disposal of waste products. Here is how it works. The venioles are a hydrophilic tube—hydrophilic means water-loving or water-attracting. When you place a hydrophilic tube in bulk water (regular water), it creates a flow of that water. This is perpetual motion. This happens because the hydrophilic tube nature of the venioles creates a layer of structured water, lining the tube, and the blood being like bulk water causes a voltage, resulting in work or the circulation of blood upward and back to the veins and heart. This is an exact and intricate design that totally changes how we look at the heart and the entire human body. For a more in-depth explanation, I encourage you to read Gerald Pollock and Thomas Cowan's work.

A term called *memory transference* has been coined to depict the act of a heart transplant recipient having memories of events not in their own, but in the organ donor's life. Paul P. Pearsall illustrated this. He tells a story of a white, middle-aged man, who worked all his life in a factory and had racist beliefs. He never in his life listened to classical or opera music. After he had a heart transplant from an anonymous donor, his wife noticed very strange changes in his personality. He started hanging out in places mostly frequented by African Americans, and he became friends with African Americans at work. He walked differently, and he started secretly listening to classical music, especially the violin. He hid these changes for fear of the unknown, for fear of who or what he was becoming. Eventually he embraced the changes and became deeply curious about his new personality. He and his wife investigated the donor of his new heart. They learned that the heart he received came from a young African American male who had been shot and killed while walking to school. They were even more stunned to find out, years later, that the school the heart donor was walking toward was a music academy, where he was studying the violin and dreaming of becoming a classical violinist.

The amazing abilities of the heart are much more fathomable thanks to the astounding research of the Heart Math Institute. According to their research, the heart has about 40,000 sensory neurons that relay information from what the heart receives from the field back up to the brain. These neurons have both short- and long-term memory, and they send information to the brain that affects our emotional experiences. This helps us understand the amazing stories of transplant patients experiencing memory transference.

The Heart Math Institute performed a study in which they showed the amazing capabilities of the heart's intelligence. The participants in the study were connected to various sensors to measure their brainwaves, heartbeat, heart rate variability and so on. Then the participants were exposed to various images. Some images were high-arousal images, such as a snake striking or a car accident, and some were low-arousal, such as a bunny rabbit or flowers. The participants were asked to push the left mouse button. When the button was pushed, they saw a blank computer screen for six seconds, and then the computer randomly selected one of the photographs, either high-or low-arousal, and it displayed it for three seconds. After the random image appeared, the screen went blank for 10 seconds during which the computer would then prompt them to push the mouse button again for the next image. They repeated this protocol about 30 times.

After the Heart Math Institute analyzed all the data, they were astounded by the results. What they found was that the heart seemed to know the images before the participants ever saw the images with their own eyes. If the picture to be projected was one of the high-arousal photos, the heart rate would drop about five seconds before the image showed on the screen. There is no way the participants would know what this picture was going to be. In the time before the image was shown, the heart rate had a much greater deceleration if the image was going to be a high-arousal image. In the calming low-arousal images, there was no significantly decelerated heart rate.

What they concluded was the heart actually knows before something in the third dimensional world happens. The heart picks up the information from the field and sends it to the brain, where the brain then has a response and sends the information back to the body. After all this, then the body will have a physical response. This response could be a feeling in the gut or the hair on the back of your neck standing up. This is another example of the pattern of input-process-output. At the point when the information becomes conscious to us, the real flow of information has already been picked up by the heart from the quantum field several seconds, in fact, before the actual event occurs in our consciousness.

What this body of research is telling us is that the heart seems to be connected to a type of intuition not bound by the limits of time or space. What is this source of intuition, and how can we learn to tap into more of this? This is the field of energy we have been discussing in the entirety of this book. This field is not bound by space and time and is filled with limitless information. Remember what Einstein said, that this field is the sole governing agent of the particle. This means that all our physical experience, everything, is being created by this One Source.

Starting from the first energy center and working our way up, as we start tuning into our heart space behind our sternum, we ingrain the coherence of the information to our brain and body. We become more connected, and we start living with more trust because we now know this invisible energy is real. And the only certainty of it is that it is love.

Heart coherence is simply the constructive interference or good vibes gaining rhythm and therefore momentum. As we practice generating the good vibes, the body has no choice but to raise its energy. The vibrational interference is growing because of its coherence. Now our brain becomes more orderly and coherent, further influencing this constructive interference of love and washes through our entire body. It heals, strengthens and uplifts our body to its natural state. This momentum is now picked up by everyone around us, and they too will entrain their energies to match this frequency if we continually practice.

## Cervical Spine. Neck

Now that our heart is open, we must put our head on straight, and there is no better way to do that than through our neck. If we are living in the slumped, rounded shoulders and forward-leaning head posture, our neck is not centered on top of our body. This causes extra strain and tension through all the neck's vertebrae, muscles and ligaments. Over time, the imbalance of this posture combined with overflow of the stress hormones of cortisol and adrenaline, we end up with a pain, injury or tension headache we just cannot figure out. We go get massaged, popped, taped, ultra-sounded, electric stemmed and Thera-Gunned, yet the pain keeps coming back. We buy a new pillow, a new bed, a new couch, a new desk. We try everything, but our neck still hurts. What gives?

Hopefully, I have created enough of an understanding for you to know by now. We must change our state and therefore our energy, and we must get our head on straight (i.e., bring our head back and over our body in the proper anatomical position). As you can see in Figure 21, there is a very strong pull on the muscles of the neck with a forward head posture, especially the sternocleidomastoid and upper trapezius. This imbalance and improper length-tension relationship of these muscles can lead to a wide variety of pains and dysfunctions.

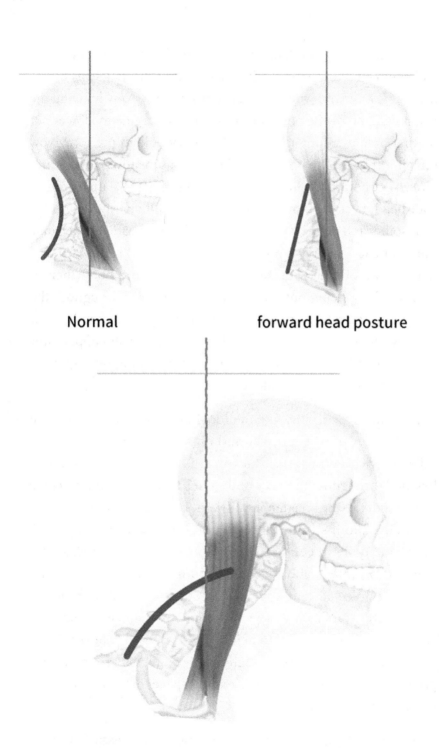

Normal                    forward head posture

*Figure 21*

Imagine a semi-bendable six-foot pole with a very heavy round ball connected to the top of it. Imagine that this pole was firmly held at its base and would not move from there. Now imagine the ball on the top of the pole moving. Can you imagine the forces put on that pole to counter balance the heavy ball on the top? Now imagine that the heavy ball at the top was steady and still and directly on top of the pole without swaying. This is analogous to your head, neck and the rest of your spine. Obviously, the pole is your spine, and the heavy ball at the top is your head. The average human head weighs 12 pounds. When the head is forward and not in a plumb line with the rest of the spine and body, there is a strong force being put on the neck and spine. Throughout the entire day, these tensions and forces are being dealt with by your spine without you even knowing. Think of what will happen over time even without the hormones of stress pumping through your body and just these forces alone.

Now imagine if, just like the ideal posture in Figure 21 you brought your head back over and on top of your body. This is called cervical retraction. Can you see how the forces would be lessened throughout the neck and spine? It is a very simple yet life changing fix. Now imagine if you went down the line of the postural checkpoints from there. While holding your head back over your body in cervical retraction, now pull your shoulder blades down, back and together opening your heart. Contract your core brace, locking your ribcage down, you pull your tummy in engaging your transverse abdominus, you squeeze your butt cheeks and tilt your pelvis to neutral, and you pull your perineum up and in. Be careful—you might just levitate you are so decompressed. This is levity. You are creating space, order and balance everywhere in your body.

To practice cervical retraction, you might find it easier to lay on your back with your knees bent and a comfortable pillow if you

208

need one. You may not like a pillow. You are the one who will know best as you now know how to listen to what your body is telling you. In supine, practice retracting your head back and down into the pillow without causing pain or discomfort. Find the sweet spot. And when you do, add the rest of the postural checkpoints to this.

When combining everything together, you may notice this causes pain or discomfort in different areas of your body. This is ok. You obviously do not want to continue with the pain and discomfort, so simply adjust the contraction levels of different postural checkpoints until you find the sweet spot. The sweet spot is coherent. It is the rhythm you are looking for. You want to pursue the sweet spot or the pain-free zone. As you practice this again and again, you will find that the pain goes away more and more.

As you find the sweet spot in laying down in supine with your knees bent, work your way to sitting and now work on engaging all the postural checkpoints in the sitting position. Then progress to standing, all the while staying in your sweet spot without pain. Note that when the postural checkpoints are done in different positions, their pain or discomfort may shift. This is ok. Remember, listen to the pain and readjust to what it tells you. The pressures of the spine are changing and pushing on different nerves, compressing different tissues and shifting pressures around. Continue working to find the sweet spot as you move into different positions.

To find variations and additional movements while holding the postural checkpoints go to casonlehman.com/wth for video tutorials.

## Fifth Energy Center. Thyroid Gland

The thyroid gland sits in the front of the neck just on top of our trachea or wind pipe. This is the home of the fifth energy center.

It is slightly below and superficial to the voice box. This gland is responsible for the production of hormones T3 (triiodothyronine) and T4 (thyroxine). These hormones play an important role in metabolism, the regulation of our weight, energy levels, internal temperature, skin, hair and nail growth and more.

Now that we have established a firm base of knowing who we are and established our creative energy of the first center we move this energy to the second center where we feel the safety and security of truly being honest with who we are. We then move this combined energy to the third center of standing strong in our own personal power of our true self, now we bring this energy up and into the heart where we feel the utmost amount of love for our precious life. Our heart blossoms and opens like a flower blooming, and now this energy moves up into our fifth energy center where we express how much love for life we have. This is the energy center to express our truth. We express how we actually feel and are not ashamed of it. This enriches our love for life even more because we are being exactly who we want to be. We shout it from the roof tops, for we are proud to be our unique selves.

## Sixth Energy Center. The Pineal Gland

The pineal gland sits in the center of the brain above the throat in the central and posterior aspect of the brain. It is housed between the right and left hemispheres of the brain in a central space that yogic masters of old called the cave of Brahma. The pineal gland is no bigger than a grain of rice. This is what mystics of antiquity have called the third eye. And rightfully so, as we now know that the pineal gland tissue has rods and cones just as our eye does. However, because it does not get direct light from our physical environment, it sits very deep in the center of the brain, when activated, it picks up or "sees" if you will, the invisible electromagnetic information from the field. It also is receiving information from the retina based on the light it receives from the environment controlling our sleep and wakeful states.

If you remember the light spectrum (refer to page ?), you will remember that what the rods and cones of our eye pick up is less than 1% of the actual light around us. Light is energy and energy is expressed in waves. The pineal gland is a transducer or a receiver and is able to pick up this information from the field around us. Just as an antenna picks up information from the field and turns it into images on a screen, the pineal gland has the same capabilities. The pineal gland is a primary input device.

The pineal picks this information up via its unique hexagonal-shaped calcite crystals embedded in it. Through vibration, these crystals pick up or download the energy from the field and turn this information into images or experiences in our mind's eye. Just like a television is able to take information it is receiving and turn it into a picture show on its screen. As we get beyond our analytical mind, and the heart and brain are in perfect coherence, we are able to tap into this intelligence that defies our perception of space and time. As the pineal gland becomes activated, these experiences we are capable of having are very mystical. They are beyond our three-dimensional space and time and often described as other worldly. These occurrences are so real that many people often describe them as leaving their physical bodies and having very real experiences of alternate spaces and times. These are called transcendental experiences.

If you have ever looked through a kaleidoscope, you have seen sacred geometric shapes, patterns and colors. This is what many have described seeing as their pineal is activated. As the pineal gland and our mind decode this information, it is often described as resembling intricate geometric patterns or fractals. The beauty of this experience we witness is often beyond the ability to describe with words.

Everyone's experience is unique and indescribable. Whatever the information may be that the pineal gland is able to pick up, our mind has the amazing ability to descramble and decode this information and turn it into profound imagery. In this transcendental moment, we are able to have the most real sensory experience without actually doing anything in the three-dimensional world. This experience is so life changing that many have had to stay in bed for days while their autonomic nervous system recalibrated. They often describe feeling amounts of love they did not know were possible to have. The people now see through the veil of the material world and are connected to the wholeness and oneness of the universe. The menial stresses that used to bother them no longer do as they see from a much higher state of consciousness.

The imagery of fractals humans see via the pineal gland during this transcendental experience is seen in the divine order of nature all around us. This has sparked the interest of many scientists and mathematicians to study these patterns. Fractals and the mathematics of them are being studied by many quantum physicists. Fractal patterns can be seen everywhere in nature. Fibonacci's sequence is one pattern of sacred geometry we see all around us. Take a look at Figure 22 to see the unfolding of the mathematics of this golden ration. For instance, this mathematical order can be seen in a pine cone or a snail shell. What this points to is astounding. We can see and recognize patterns from the mathematics of the fractals. This shows us that the invisible field of intelligence is magnificently ordered into our three-dimensional world and shows us its form through mathematics. As we open our focus and become more aware of the world around us, we can see more and more of the divine order within it. Refer to Figures 22-25 to see the connection of how this ratio is tied to nature.

## The Fibonacci Sequence

1,1,2,3,5,8,13,21,34,55,89,144,233,377...

| | |
|---|---|
| $1+1=2$ | $8+13=21$ |
| $1+2=3$ | $13+21=34$ |
| $2+3=5$ | $21+34=55$ |
| $3+5=8$ | $34+55=89$ |
| $5+8=13$ | $55+89=144$ |

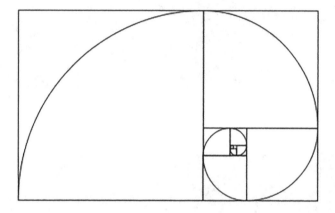

*Figure 22*

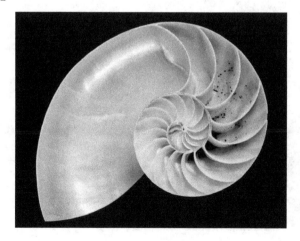

*Figure 23*

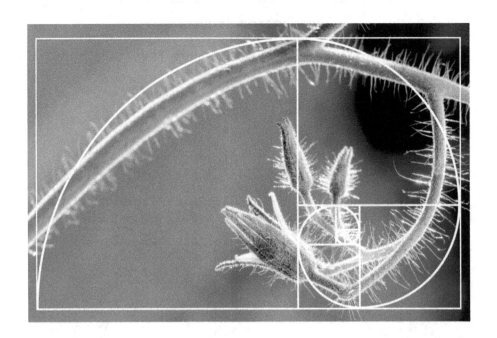

*Figure 24*

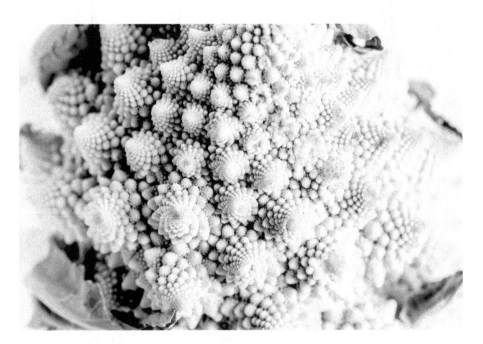

*Figure 25*

It is very interesting that it has been estimated that the pineal glands of up to 80% of Americans are calcified. This calcification is said to be due to the toxicity of our environment, specifically the toxicity of our food and water. We will talk about dietary practices to decalcify in the next section. It is also very interesting that the pineal gland has its crystals fully intact when we are first born. Many children around the approximate ages of four to nine recall having mystical experiences where they see fractal patterns and have lucid dreams beyond their body recalling the experiences vividly. The child's brain is not yet analytical, so information coming in is much less analyzed and more real. This makes a lot of sense now that we know there is an infinite amount of information available in the field all the time. Children naturally pick this information up. Often this magnificence is shunned by many societal influences calling it silly, not real and unaccepted. This causes the child to believe that this is silly and not real, and they no longer give their attention to these experiences in order to be socially accepted and not cast out.

The pineal gland is quite simply out of this world as you can see from above, and to understand its superpowers to a greater degree we must learn about its biochemical function. The pineal gland is the endocrine gland responsible for the production of melatonin and serotonin. You may have heard of these two very popular hormones. Serotonin is believed to be largely responsible for our mood regulation. Remember that a large part of serotonin is also made in the EEC in the intestines as well. This points to an even deeper gut-brain axis.

Melatonin is most commonly known for its benefits of making us sleepy, however, as we study this amazing hormone more in depth, we are learning some fascinating things about it. As we perceive light or dark through our retina, the optic nerve stimulates the suprachiasmatic nuclei in our brain. This is known as our biological clock, and it helps set the rhythms of all the organs of our body. From here through a chain of biochemical reactions, the pineal gland is stimulated via a neurotransmitter called norepinephrine. The overall purpose here is to cause the amino acid tryptophan to convert into serotonin and then convert the serotonin into melatonin.

When the sun goes down and it gets dark, melatonin production goes up. As we become sleepier, our brainwaves change from a beta brainwave frequency into a slower alpha frequency, and this is where we slip into our nightly sleep. As we drift away, we then fall into an even deeper theta frequency where we dream and have creative insights. When we sleep, we experience an altered state of consciousness. Remember, the same happens during meditation as we fall into alpha and theta brainwaves when our analytical mind is quieted. During meditation, however, as we practice, we stay right in the sweet spot between wakefulness and sleep. This is between the brainwave states of alpha, theta and delta. During deep and restorative sleep, we are in the delta brainwave state. Finally, gamma brainwaves are found when humans enter a flow state or have a transcendental experience. Refer back to figure 5 on page ?? to review the brain waves.

Melatonin is at its peak between 1:00 a.m. and 4:00 a.m. during our altered state of consciousness of sleep. In darkness, as melatonin is released into the brain and body, some amazing things happen. It turns out there are many amazing chemicals derived from melatonin, and this all happens by our body's own intelligence. Melatonin gets biologically advanced into powerful chemicals by our body alone. One of its derivatives is a phosphorescent bioluminescent molecule. This makes sense, because as the pineal gland activates, we see amazing vivid colors as in a fractal kaleidoscope. Another one of its metabolites is the popular hallucinogenic known as DMT (dimethyl-5-methoxy-triptamine). DMT has been coined the spirit molecule by Rick Strassman. It is widespread throughout the plant kingdom. This powerful molecule is responsible for the out of body and near-death experiences many times described in the transcendental moments. For thousands of years, the shamans have used a sacred formula from plants to make a drink called ayahuasca, which allows them to see beyond the confines of this three-dimensional world and tap into the clairvoyance of the Universe. The plants ayahuasca is made from have the powerful DMT molecule in them. Another derivative of melatonin is the sedative called benzodiazepine, pharmaceutically known as Valium and Xanax. This allows the body to feel zero pain or discomfort, making the mystical experience the most comfortable feeling one ever had. This is all done with the body's innate intelligence.

Melatonin is very important in our overall health too. When the body has an experience like the aforementioned transcendental moments, our body receives a biological upgrade and coherence, and order follows suit. However, it is not just by having a transcendental moment that we receive its benefits. As we practice balancing and sustaining our attention on all our energy centers, the entire body works more rhythmically, thus creating better balance in total hormone production. This allows melatonin to do the same, and now the circadian rhythms of all our organs are in better alignment, allowing the body to create its natural state of health. We will learn more about our body's circadian rhythms and more techniques to help realign our body's rhythms in the next section. However, the practice of placing our attention on all our energy centers is one of the best ways to improve our body's circadian rhythms.

When melatonin is present, cortisol goes down. This means we are not stressing. It lowers triglyceride levels. It reduces atherosclerosis or hardening of the arteries since this is a side effect of cortisol. It pumps up the immune system and promotes DNA repair. It improves carbohydrate metabolism to lower our blood glucose levels.

## Seventh Energy Center. Pituitary Gland

This energy center is located in the center of your head. The pituitary gland is known as *the master gland*. This is the head of the household—it manages and regulates all hormonal glands in the body. In the pattern of input, processing, output, the pituitary gland is the output as it governs and leads the rest of the glands, much like a head coach would lead her team. As the pineal gland receives the information from the field, the signal passes through the third ventricle of the brain. This signal is processed by the hypothalamus and the thalamus, and then this processed information is sent to the pituitary gland, the master gland, where this information is sent throughout the body to coordinate the body's functions.

As the pineal gland activates and sends instructions to the pituitary gland, the latter releases two awesome chemicals called oxytocin and vasopressin. You may have heard of oxytocin as the love hormone and for good reason. In mammals, oxytocin is the chemical responsible for the bonding between a mother and her offspring. After birth, the mother releases oxytocin into her bloodstream to create a loving connection with her babies to ensure that her offspring will have a life-sustaining connection to better the survival of the species. A similar release of oxytocin is present in human mothers and their children when the baby exits the birth canal and is first held by the mother. This marks the unconditional love a mother has for her child.

When oxytocin is secreted by the pituitary gland, it causes nitrous oxide to open the flood gates of blood into the heart. Remember that the derived endothelial relaxing factor allow for the heart literally to swell with love. This is present during a transcendental experience as well. Along with the release of oxytocin and the profound increase in heart energy, the pituitary releases a hormone called vasopressin. This is an antidiuretic hormone. What this means is when this hormone is in higher amounts in the body, it causes the kidneys and therefore the body to retain water. Now with more water in the blood, the body becomes an even stronger conductor for electricity, allowing every cell in our body to get an increase in energy from the unified field.

The seventh energy center is also known as the center for oneness of all creation. This is our center for unbounded awareness, where we see beyond space and time. This is the energy center of our divinity. When this center is open and active, we have clarity of our purpose on this planet. We have alignment with the higher consciousness of source energy, and we feel whole and complete.

## Eighth Energy Center. You and the Universe

This is the only energy center we will learn about in this book which is not part of our physical body. This energy center is located anywhere from a few inches to about 16 inches above our head. It is our connection to the Universe, God or the unified field of energy that we are. This energy center is a symbol of our eternal self as it stays with us forever and is not within our physical body. As you become more aware of the seven energy centers in and around your body, the eighth center will intensify.

Personally, it feels like the branch of a tree is tickling the top of my head, and as I place my attention on it, I can feel the energy radiating up above my crown. This center was called the Ka by the Egyptians and was illustrated in paintings as a halo around the head of Christ, Buddha and other religious figures.

## Our Energetic Body. The Torus Field

A torus is a donut shaped three-dimensional field of moving energy. This moving field of energy revolves bidirectionally from top to bottom and bottom to top. Think of a donut folding in on itself continually, revolving back around in a three-dimensional spherical fashion. Refer to Figure 25 to see the toroidal field around our body. This toroidal energy field continually exists around everything: people, trees, the earth, sun and the universe. If you have ever heard someone say a person has a nice aura to them, then this aura is our toroidal field. Some very intuitive humans are able to see colors or energies around other human beings. This field of energy is connecting us with everything and everyone at all times. Just as the electron cloud floats around the atom until consciousness is placed upon it (the observer effect), we too have an aura or energetic field around us. We are just trillions upon trillions of those electron clouds of the atom coalescing into matter. This makes our field much larger. And the coolest thing is that we have the power through metacognition to make our field grow. By becoming aware that we command the ability to be aware of our energy centers and then by putting our loving intention for the greatest good of each of those centers, we create more coherence and health in each of the cells of the individual centers. When practicing this repeatedly, our field and subsequent coherence of that field develop within and around us.

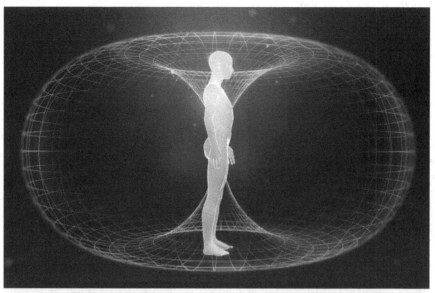

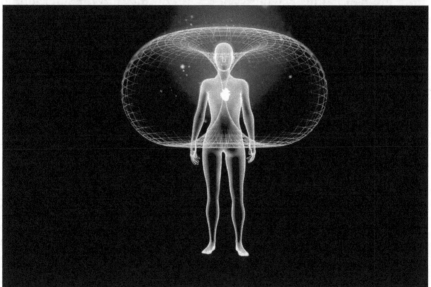

*Figure 25*

Our heart has the strongest toroidal field in our body. This is the electromagnetic field that is measurable up to nine feet away. Each individual energy center has this toroidal flow moving around it. Each energy center has its own field, and this energy can be in varying degrees of strength depending on the health and coherence of the individual energy center. These fields of energy within us and all around us are not in a fixed shape. They move and wobble as we are more or less in energetic rhythm, alignment and coherence. And the universal energy from the earth, other humans and groups of humans plays into this dynamic field of energy. As the seven energy centers become attuned with each other, working into increased coherence, the torus field of energy around our body magnifies up and into the eighth center. Many people can feel a presence of energy above their head around the eighth energy center. This is the top of the toroidal field, where I mentioned I feel like a tree branch is tickling my head. This is where energy is coming into the energetic body of us. This energy works down into the energy of the earth and then back around. Again, in both directions, one spiraling upward and the other spiraling downward.

Konstantin Korotkov has developed a methodology to measure this invisible field of energy around and in our bodies. By using a technology called gas discharge visualization (GDV), the strength or weakness of the field around our body and the energy centers within our body can be measured, giving us extremely beneficial feedback to make changes in our personal energy fields. When we are stuck in the realm of the third dimension focusing on matter, we lose connection with the invisible field of energy all around us. We believe it only exists if we can see it with our physical eyes, touch it with our hands, hear it with our ears, taste it or smell it. However, we are tricked into the belief that what we can sense with our senses is it and only it. In the conventional medicine world, we use diagnostic tools such as MRI, EKG, EEG and more that are actually reading the electromagnetic field of the body to assess its matter, but we do not give any credit to the actual invisible electromagnetic field. We just focus our attention on the matter emitting it. But with this technology of GDV, we are now able to see with our eyes the invisible field of energy we are emitting. This allows us to learn what part of our physical body we need to focus our attention on to create more coherence and health, and then see the energetic correspondence. In the image below you can see the healthy luminous energy field compared to an unhealthy field of energy on the right. Check out Figure 26 to see a real image of a GDV measurement of a healthy versus unhealthy energy field around the person.

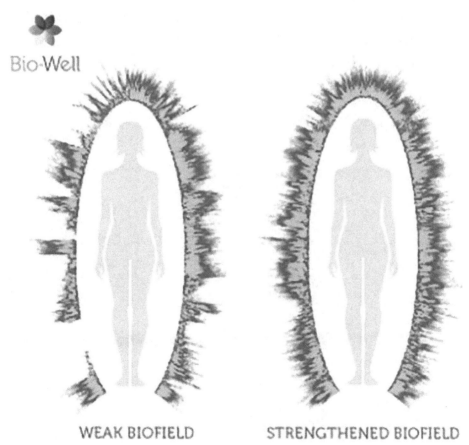

Bio-Well

WEAK BIOFIELD        STRENGTHENED BIOFIELD

*Figure 26*

## Cerebrospinal Fluid

The cerebrospinal fluid (CSF) is a clear fluid that bathes the brain and the spinal cord. It essentially keeps the brain and spinal cord floating in its liquid substance. The brain and the spine are the home of our central nervous system. It occupies the cavities within the brain called the ventricles, and it also covers the outside of the brain. Take a look at Figure 27 to see how the CSF floats and bathes the brain tissue. It travels down the central canal of the spinal cord, which is the center of the cord as well as all the way around the outside of the spinal cord, keeping the spinal cord surrounded by its fluid. The spinal cord stops at the second lumbar vertebrae, however, the CSF continues into what is called the Dural sack all the way to S2, which is in our sacrum very near our first energy center.

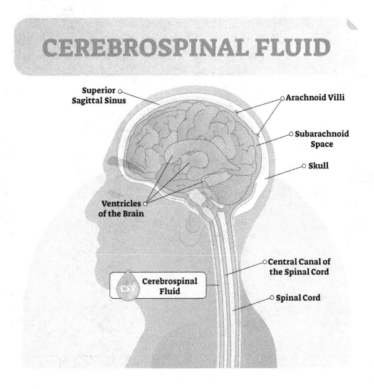

CEREBROSPINAL FLUID

*Figure 27*

At any moment during the day, we have 150 ml of CSF flowing through our spine and brain, however, we make 450-600 ml of CSF a day. This is fascinating because the CSF is so enriching that our body must replenish and renew its supply all day long. This fluid carries vital information in it, sending signals of information back and forth from the brain to the body and body to brain, all happening faster than the speed of light. This means it is happening on a quantum level. It transports nutrients and hormones to the central nervous system. It instructs stem cells to proliferate or differentiate. Proliferation means that a cell can reproduce and make more of whatever it needs to replenish. Differentiate means a cell can morph into whatever the body needs it to become for the overall good of our health. We are superhuman, and we may not even know it.

Stem cells are specialized cells that have the ability to turn into any kind of cell the body needs. In today's medical world, there are loads of research being done on stem cells. Many doctors are specializing in stem-cell therapy where they inject stem cells harvested from either the patient's own adipose tissue or bone marrow into a part of the body that needs healing. Our CSF has the ability already built in for the proliferation and differentiation of these stem cells. But when living by the hormones of stress, having poor posture and improper nutrition, we are not being gifted the maximum potential of the magnificence our body has to offer. Our CSF flow is altered, and the energetics the proper flow of it creates throughout our body has glitches in it. This slump causes incoherence, lowering our overall systemic energy.

Conversely, when we are living in the state of love, and we are grounded in our truth, holding our posture in the tone of greatness, the CSF's magical capabilities come back online. As a fluid flow returns to the CSF, it now becomes a receiver and transmitter of energy vibration and information. With its all-encompassing connections to the entire central nervous system, it is able to instruct our body into its regenerative abilities beyond our current understanding.

Just as Masaru Emoto's experiments with water show that water is able to transmit the feelings of love, joy and peace through its intricate fractal pattern creations, so too can the CSF absorb, store and transmit the essence of the unified field within us and all around us into and throughout our human body.

Now let us gain an understanding of where the CSF is stored inside the brain. We know it surrounds the brain, but the areas inside the brain in which it connects are fascinating. As you can see by looking at Figure 28, the inner ventricles of the brain create a connection to all sections of the brain. Take a look at the lateral ventricle and notice how it makes contact with the frontal lobe, the occipital lobe, the parietal lobe and also has a projection in the rear of the brain to have a connection with the visual sensory area of the brain. The CSF also goes down into the temporal lobe where the hippocampus lives. This is not by consequence but rather through elegant creation as these ventricles are allowing instant messages at quantum speed to be relayed through the cerebrospinal fluid to all aspects of the brain and the entire body. Making every one of us a collective whole unit of oneness that achieves total synchronization and coordinates all bodily and brain functions simultaneously beyond our understanding of space and time.

# Ventricular system

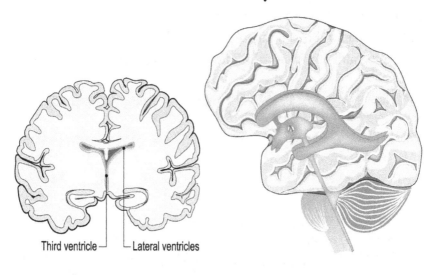

Third ventricle — Lateral ventricles

*Figure 28*

We also must take a closer look at the third ventricle of the brain in more depth, as therein lies a captivating design. In the anterior peak of the third ventricle, it connects with the pituitary gland, and the posterior peak connects directly with the pineal gland, the home of our seventh and sixth energy centers. Going back to the pineal gland being the primary manufacturer of melatonin, there is very good evidence that the CSF is the primary distribution method of this potent health-promoting chemical throughout the entire brain and body. DMT, the spirit molecule and a derivative of melatonin, has been found at some of its highest concentrations in the CSF compared to other fluids of the body. As you can see by looking at Figure 29, the pineal gland sits just on the back wall of the third ventricle, and the pituitary sits on the front of the third ventricle. This is the house of the third eye, or what many yogic traditions called the cave of Brahma. Daoist's have called this area of the brain the crystal palace. Here in this center of the brain is where the spiritual world turns into the physical world. Imagine the cerebral spinal fluid from Figures 27 and 28 bathing the inside and outside of the brain as a perfect vehicle to deliver melatonin and all other vital nutrients to our entire brain and body, working as a fluid conductor to transmit health throughout our entire body.

# PINEAL GLAND

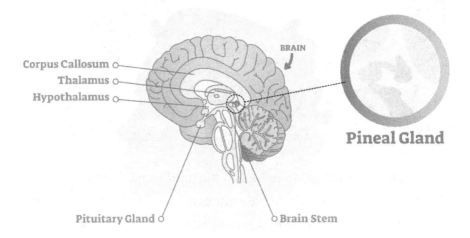

Figure 29

As we change our state of being and align our posture into its correlating position of the greatest version of ourself, CSF begins to biologically upgrade. By engaging our postural checkpoints, we are creating space in our vertebrae, allowing CSF to regain its energetic flow. This flow allows the CSF to work its magic, increasing the proliferation of stem cells. By simply placing our attention on each individual energy center for two to four minutes, starting with one and working our way up to eight, we are following the path of this sacred fluid creating a vortex of energy all the way up and down our central canal. This creates even more upgrades to this fluid bathing and detoxifying all the fog out of our

228

brain and spine. We are vibrant, fresh, clean and open to a brand-new outlook on life.

You now have the knowledge of the foundational checkpoints of your entire body's postural health. You have learned how to contract and engage these muscles and their correlation and causation of flow of pathologies throughout the entire body. Starting with the first postural checkpoint, the muscles of the pelvic floor all the way up to the top, cervical retraction, you now have a better understanding of how to structurally hold your body to regain its maximal biomechanical function. In addition to this structural foundation, you now understand and can practice embodying the energy centers of your body. Understanding these sacred centers by knowing where they are in the body and the hormonal function, as well as its basic biochemical purpose, you further your neural network of knowledge to catapult you into facing the ego's attempt to talk you out of change.

## Awakening the Chakras/ Energy Centers Meditation

Get comfortable in your meditation chair and eliminate all distractions. Either use the meditation music you have already chosen, or you can search specifically for chakra meditation music. Whatever inspires you. You can search on the Internet for many choices of the chakra/energy center meditations that are guided, telling you where to place your attention, which may suit you. Also, there are many specifically made songs where the music rhythms change for each chakra/energy center where you are focusing in and around. This is a great choice if you would like to do this meditation on your own. Play around with all that is available at your fingertips on the Internet and find a style that suits you. The act of practicing this meditation is all that matters.

To begin, close your eyes, take a few deep breaths, and slow your breathing. Calm yourself and find your center. Relax. And then relax even more, letting go of the tension in your neck and body.

Remember the intention of this meditation is to keep your conscious attention on each individual energy center as well as you can. In doing so, you are directing matter (cells and molecules) to work in greater order. This creates coherence and rhythm, which then creates health. Where your attention goes, your energy flows!

Now put all your attention and focus on the first energy center in your perineum. To help bring your focus to this area, squeeze the muscles of the pelvic floor. Keep your focus on this area more and more. If your mind starts to drift, bring your attention back to this area and focus again, more intently on this area. Do this for about two minutes. Now broaden your focus to the area of space around this first center. This is very different because this is not part of your physical body, but the point here is to place your attention on the wave function of this center. It helps me to imagine a beach ball circumference around my perineum and hips. Remember, this is the invisible field of energy that this chakra or energy wheel is emitting into the field. For the first energy center, you want to place your attention around your hips and inner thighs so you can imagine this beach ball around your pelvis. Practice feeling this space around your body. Remember, this is a divergent focus. After about a minute or so of divergently focusing on the wave or field of energy around the first energy center, bring your attention back convergently to your first center and love all the work the cells in it are doing for you, sending this center your best intentions for coherence and order.

As you feel your energy in your first center convergently, purposefully move your attention and focus up to the second energy center. This is the space just behind your naval and down an inch or two. It does not have to be an exact science, so focus on your naval is just fine. Bring all your awareness to this area. Again, keep your focus here for about two minutes and practice bringing your attention back to this space if your mind wanders. Every time you bring your focus back is a victory. Now take your focus divergently in the space outside your body around your belly button. Feel this space around your second center and stay there for a minute. Practice feeling the energy you cannot see but that you can feel with your awareness. Here again, for the difficult to grasp novelty of the divergent focus, I find it helps to think of a hula hoop floating around my waist to feel the energy of space around me. Now bring your attention convergently back to your second center in your body and send it all your love. Being so grateful for all the enzymatic reactions it creates in order for you to digest and use the food you eat for your body's nourishment.

Take this combined energy from your first and second energy center and bring it up with your intent focus to your third energy center in the pit of your gut, just below the Xiphoid Process of your sternum. This is your center of personal power and self-esteem. Feel this energy in the pit of your gut and focus all your attention on it for two minutes, bringing your attention back if your mind wanders. After two minutes, take your attention and focus it divergently to the space around this third chakra and tap into the energy around your third center. Focus on this space outside your physical body for one minute. Now bring your focus back to your physical body in your third energy center and love these adrenal glands for balancing their hormone production for the greatest good of your entire body. Thank the cells and tissues of this third center for all the work they do behind the scenes. Take your power back and give it to yourself.

Take this powerful energy from the combination of the first, second and third energy centers and raise it right up and into your heart! There is nothing more powerful than love. Feel your heart open. Feel the love of life light up your fourth energy center. Bask in this energy and feel the love for life. Enjoy it and relax into this feeling. This is the center with the largest electromagnetic field, measurable up to nine feet away from your body. Feel the power of love within your fourth center. Keep your focus and attention here for two minutes and then practice feeling the space divergently around your heart. Imagine the walls of the room you are in and see if you can feel your heart's energy flowing out toward them. Practice intently feeling this energy around your body. Feel it on either side of your shoulders at the level of your heart and see if you can even feel it directly behind your heart, in the space behind your back. I like to think of the rings of Saturn orbiting around my heart center, extending them out as far as I can. Now bring your attention and focus back to the space where your heart lives behind your sternum and give thanks to all this amazing organ does for you. Feel gratitude for it automatically functioning and giving you life. Keeping you alive without you having to do anything. This is truly amazing!

Now all the combined energy from the first through fourth centers work up into the fifth energy center in the middle of your throat. The increasing frequency of energy coming up through the first four centers will be unmistakable in your throat. Often, I feel this energy coming out of my mouth as I breathe out. This is your voice. This is your self-expression. This is how you speak your truth. Feel this energy in your throat for two minutes and bring your attention back to it if it slips away. After about two minutes, feel this energy in the space around your neck outside your body again like the rings orbiting around the planet Saturn. Feel the invisible space. After one minute, bring your attention and focus back to your fifth center in your throat and thank it for all it does for you. All the thyroid functions. Your ability to speak your mind and say what is on your heart. All of it. Give it your loving attention.

Now, from five, you will take your energy to six, the pineal gland. This is the space in the back of your head just above and behind the beginning of your throat. Picture the gland in your head and bring your focus to it. Feel that spot in your head where it sits. Feel the combined energy from your body's five energy centers rising into your pineal gland. Keep your focus here for two minutes, and then broaden your focus to the space around your head, like waves rippling out from the pineal gland. Again, in the pineal gland, I like to focus all the way around my head as far out as I can go. I think of a blinking electrical tower sending its radar way out and around into the field of energy to see what it can pick up. Remember, the pineal gland is a transducer and picks up the information all around you in the field. After a minute or so of feeling the space around the pineal gland in your head, draw your focus convergently back to the sixth center in your brain. Give this part of your body love and gratitude for all the amazing functions it does without you even knowing. Feel the energy in that center.

Now take the combined energy in the pineal gland and with your focus and intention take this energy to the middle of your brain, the seventh energy center. This is the pituitary gland. Remember the pituitary is the leader of all the glands, synchronizing the order and operation of the brain and the body. Feel this! All the energy from one through seven coming up and into the seventh center in the middle of your brain. Focus your attention here for two minutes and then take your focus divergently outside of your head and around it. Feel the space on either side of your head and then feel the space in front and back of your head. As if you were wearing a sombrero hat, imagine the space all the way around your head. Feel it! This is energy. Now after about a minute of that, bring your attention and focus back to the center of your head. Give your pituitary gland love for orchestrating the infinitesimal amounts of functions throughout your body. As you do this, feel your body respond to this love.

Bring your focus and attention to the space six inches above your head. This is the eighth energy center. Feel the sensation of energy above your head and focus intently on this area for two minutes. Feel how this energy is moving down into your head like a vortex. Imagine a three-dimensional waterfall, flowing down and into your head. This energy center is the top of the toroidal field you have around you, always. Because you have generated so much coherent energy, you can now feel this flowing field torus around you and flowing through you. There is no need to take your attention divergently around this center because you already are focusing your attention divergently. Keep your focus here for about two minutes or so. While your attention is here, practice feeling gratitude for this amazing experience. Enjoy the wonderful feeling and be grateful for it.

Now divergently feel the space around your entire body. Feel the energy flowing around you. Feel this for two minutes or so. Feel your body radiating with light (energy). If you did not know you are energy, now you will because you can feel it. That is energy, and it is part of you.

Now take your focus even further divergently. Go into the blackness as far as you can outside of your body. Imagine going deep into the blackness way out beyond your body. Take your focus into the field that is everything. Feel the deep sense of oneness with all that is. Relax into this magnificence of the Intelligence of all life. Let it love you. Feel the love it brings always. Feel worthy to receive its love.

Now slowly bring all that energy back to your body and slowly wiggle your hands and toes. Bring your attention to your heart and feel the love you just witnessed. Continue to bring your awareness back to your body and slowly open your eyes whenever you are ready. You might need to lie down to let the energy work into and through your nervous system. You might just want to sit in the peace of it for a while. Do whatever feels right.

Take this loving energy with you throughout your entire day.

# Section Four:
# **Food & Healing**

In this section of the book, I am not going to try and tell you I have the exact perfect diet for you. There is no such thing as a perfect diet. Actually, 80% of diets end up failing because there is no one size fits all approach. As you have learned through epigenetics, there is an infinitesimal number of outcomes that can be turned on or turned off for our health. What is coming into our mouth is just another component of the signals flowing from the environment around our cells to our genes. We have learned how our thoughts, state of being—created from our thoughts, posture and awareness of our energy centers—can all change the signal to the cell epigenetically. Now we will gain a further knowledge base of how food is another signal we are giving our body. This food can be health promoting or dis-ease promoting.

We all have different needs nutritionally. What works for me may not work for you, however, some things that have worked for me can work for you. Who knows? Realistically, you do! As namely you become the scientist of your life and increase your awareness, you will be able to understand what is working for you and what is not. What I do know is that real, whole, unprocessed food is medicine. And I also know that the ultra-processed nutritionally depleted food available to us today is not medicine. It, in fact, is poisoning us very slowly. In this section it is my intent to educate you and help you understand how food can be a springboard to get your health back to its innate capacity.

In this section, I will teach you what I call "not food," that is the highly processed, hyper-caloric food designed in a science lab, made to be irresistible. You will become better educated on how and why this food is highly addictive while adding to our body's overall stress via inflammation. We will understand how food works with our health epigenetically. I will teach you about intermittent fasting and how it plays into our circadian rhythms as well as gaining a firm understanding of what our circadian rhythms are. Finally, I will give you some very broad and basic health promoting foods and what foods to stay away from.

Before we dive into the details, I want to point out one important piece of wisdom I have learned on my personal journey. Food can and will have life-changing positive effects not only on your health but on your spiritual path as well. It has on mine, and it has taken my life to a whole new level. This is because my brain and body started to work properly again, and I was able to utilize more of my full creative potential. However, because of its profound change in my physical body (I lost 60 pounds) and my mental state (I no longer experienced brain fog and finally had a clear mind), I began to give food and what was for dinner all my vital lifeforce energy. In other words, I was giving my power away to food. I found myself looking down on others' food choices and making assumptions that food was what was making them sick. I also began to push my food choices on family and friends. My life revolved around reading ingredients labels. Like I said, I was feeling great. Many of my symptoms I experienced before were gone. However, some would come back every now and again.

It was not until I started studying the work of a number of scholars and began to meditate that I became conscious of the state of being I was living in. I was so passionate about food and its health-changing effects that it began to create an energetic imbalance in me. I was living in a state of fear by worrying about the ingredients in food. As I continued to meditate, I realized this. It became conscious to me that because I was in a state of anxious worry when it came to food, I was not effectively absorbing the perfect organic meal I cared so passionately about. Because of the hormones of stress, my energy was being utilized in the fight-or-flight nervous system instead of the rest and digest nervous system. No matter what diet you are eating, if you are eating it and living in a state of chronic stress, the body is going to be insufficiently absorbing whatever nutrients are in that food. As we now know, the body's energy is being transported from the gut to the large muscles of our body, heart and brain because of a perceived threat.

Aha! That was why some repeated symptoms were coming back again and again. Symptoms like neck pain and skin rashes. I realized I needed to love my gut and body for all it was doing for me. As I practiced and learned to become more conscious of placing my attention in my gut and stomach (second and third energy centers) and awaken the power of these cells, tissues and organs, I started to slowly notice a difference in my overall digestion. I learned not to be overly concerned with the ingredients of the meal because I could feel it caused my body to switch into its sympathetic nervous system. My consciousness rose to another level. I became aware of who I was being, and sure enough, the symptoms seemed to happen less and less. If any symptoms come back, I just catch who I am being and where my attention is and fix it because I know I can heal my body.

I am still very conscious of what I eat as I believe food is medicine, but it dawned on me that if I was going to stress about ingredients, then I was causing just as much dis-ease in my body as the potentially harmful food could. The point is that using food as medicine is a powerful tool but not the entire fix. If we raise our awareness and become conscious of our choices, then we have the power. And we can utilize the power in food to amplify our energy.

## The Food Industry

In order to truly make a change in the way we eat and see food, we must have some inspiration. We must wake up to what is really going on. We must gain knowledge of how the food industry plays into our psychological human instincts to manipulate us to buy their products. By learning that a few giant corporations have control over the majority of our food industry and that their singular focus is on their economic bottom line and not our health, we can see through our food addictions and take a stand not to eat the food strategically designed to be addictive. In doing so, our health will skyrocket.

Mark Hyman points out some absolutely mind-blowing statistics about the Big Food industry. In the next three paragraphs, I will paraphrase some of what he points out in his books. Just nine big food companies control what is bought and sold in all grocery stores and retail outlets in America. Yes, I said nine! These companies are the makers of seeds, agrochemicals, and Big Food companies. All these companies decide how our food is grown, what food is grown, whom the food is sold to and at what price it is sold. This locks farmers into a vicious cycle of fewer choices, less profit and more environmental damage. Recent mega mergers have allowed this control of our agriculture. Now even most of our health-food companies are owned by one of these nine big food companies.

Sixty percent of the seeds sold to farmers are controlled by only four companies. These companies are Bayer/Monsanto, ChemChina, BASF and Corverta. In 1990, there were over 100 companies that sold seeds to farmers. Today, there are only 12 plants that provide for 75% of our food, which are all controlled by these four companies. Sixty percent of these 12 plants come from corn, wheat and rice. Only three companies now control 70% of the agrochemicals used on these small amounts of commodity crops. Agrochemicals are herbicides, pesticides, insecticides, fungicides, etc. These are toxic chemicals sprayed on the crops to kill anything that can potentially eat or damage the crop's yield. These chemicals have a toxic trickle-down effect on the soil, water runoff, and the crops that eaten by humans and animals. As you can see, there is a control of our food going on. This control is not for the betterment of our health or our planet. This is all for the monetization of monocropping of mainly corn, wheat and soy. Monocropping is the practice in agriculture of only growing one crop on the same land year after year.

Genetically modified organisms (GMOs) have been developed to withstand the toxic effects of these agrochemicals. By genetically altering the seed's DNA, the mega seed companies have created a seed and crop that will not be killed by the toxic chemical spray. With no bugs, fungus, weeds, etc. to damage the growth of the crop, their yield or final product is much more profitable. Farmers have no choice but to use these genetically modified seeds and agrochemicals in order to create enough profit to sustain their livelihood. For a farmer to switch to organic seed or an entirely different crop, they would have to go through a long transition period in which the yield can fall victim to the unknown effects of Mother Nature. This is far too risky for independent farmers to take on. Many farmers are cornered into a choiceless situation.

Wheat, however, has not been genetically modified, but in 2006, the makers of Roundup found that if wheat is sprayed with their toxic chemical right before harvest, it will dry the seed out enough to keep it from developing mold when stored in silos after harvest. Therefore, being much more profitable for the farmer but lacing

240

our breads, crackers and everything wheat flour with toxic glyphosate. Consequently, we see the skyrocketing of gluten sensitivity in America starting its strong upward trend since 2006.

The extensive use of GMO's and toxic agrochemicals across America's soil creates plenty of food to be further processed for the grocery store shelves. It allows for the farmer to trust a higher yield, therefore having more financial stability. The truth is GMOs and everything that comes with them are all for profit and not health. This food system is a more than $1 trillion industry in America. It makes sense, then, that 99% of the US Government subsidies are for commodity crops like corn, wheat, soy, etc., which are further ultra-processed into the "not food," adding to our chronic disease epidemic in America. The USDA (United States Department of Agriculture) spends over $25 billion a year on subsidies. Consequently, only the remaining 1% of the 25 billion goes to farmers who grow fruits and vegetables, known as "specialty crops." It's laughable that the US government tells us to eat five to nine servings of fruits and vegetables a day. If you are a farmer and you rely on the government subsidies as a safety net of income, then it's obvious what you are cornered into farming. Now the essential vegetables we need in our diet are left in the toxic dust.

As you can see, there is an overwhelming elephant in the room we seem to be blind to as the media outlets never talk about the truth of the matter. However, because the seed has been altered from its God-given genetics, all in order to survive the manmade toxic chemicals that have to be sprayed on it to ensure its exponential profit growth, there are many downstream consequences as a result. These consequences seem to be nonchalantly swept under the rug by a very powerful few who control the information leaked to the public.

Here are some problems we have created.

## Problem # 1– Our Soil

Just as we need a rich and diverse microbiome to grow and heal into our healthiest and most vibrant selves, plants and soil need the same diversity. Plants need a wholesome balance and abundance of microbiome in their soil to thrive into nutrient dense nourishing foods. In America our soil is so deplete of minerals and nutrients that it is estimated in 60 years, if continuing to farm the way we have, our soil will be unable to grow any crops.[8] On a very large scale, our farming practices across the nation have not changed for many years causing this lack of vitality in our soil. This is due to a number of factors that the farmers of the land must conform to in order to make ends meet. Farms have had to get much bigger in order to survive and stay competitive, which has made attention to each acre of soil health much more difficult. Because of government subsidies, the farmers grow the same thing year after year, and this robs the soil of plant diversity. When the soil has plant diversity, there is a wide variety of nutrients left behind when the plants decay. This enriches the soil. Only, rotating between a few crops or no crop rotation at all (monocropping) does not give the soil enough of the variety of microbiome, which it needs to create a healthy and diverse culture. This combined with the toxic chemicals being used, which bind to the soil's microscopic natural resources, wipes out much of the biological life even further. The farmer now must put chemicals like nitrogen back into the soil after harvest because of its lifelessness.

The health of our soil comes down to three main things—making sure the soil is covered with plants at all times, diversification of what is grown, and not disrupting or tilling the soil. Cover crops are plants used as a secondary cover to give life back to the soil. These are plants like grasses, legumes or vegetables planted after the last harvest of a different crop or used between rows of crops. This allows for the increased bio-diversity to return life-sustaining nutrients and microorganisms to the soil. It creates nature's own compost pile as these crops decompose and produce different varieties of foods to eat. Bacteria and fungi decompose toxic chemicals and restore balance to the soil through their byproducts of organic matter. Due to the government only highly subsidizing corn, wheat and soy, for the farmer to choose an alternative cover crop would be a financial risk to his livelihood as well as require much more physical labor.

When we throw in the use of genetically modified seed, it is now much easier for a farmer to create a profitable yield, so there is no reason for farmers to change their practices. Combined with the government subsidies, this makes change a tough sell for farmers. This clearly is an unsustainable practice and is killing our environment and human race. The good news is Mother Earth is extremely resilient, and when regenerative farming practices are brought into the land, the soil and the amazing communication abilities of the microorganisms living in it bounce back in astonishing ways.

Be sure to buy local and support farmers who use the organic regenerate farming practices as much as you can.

## Problem # 2– Nutritionally Depleted "Not Food"

Because of the aforementioned farming practices and the genetic modification of seeds, our food has lost much of its nutrient density compared to what it should have. Our fruits and vegetables today are lacking the nutrient profile compared to 50 years ago. These commodity crops have been chosen to be mega farmed because of their relatively non-perishable, storable and transportable nature. This allows a massive part of the production to be transported throughout the world. These crops are sent via train and trucks to the milling and processing plants.

Here these crops are stripped of much of their nutrient profile while processing a very calorie rich and more palatable part of the plant. For example, grains like wheat used to be ground by a stone mill into flour, which is the base of so many things we eat, like bread. This flour consisted of the entire wheat kernel. Within this whole ground flour was all the vitamins, fiber, and other nutrients of the grain. Thanks to the industrial revolution, man-created steam mills now grind the flour. This allowed us to remove the fibrous outer bran and germ layers of the kernel, which if left in could spoil the flour. This obviously makes the flour last much longer, but it also robs the flour of protein, fat, vitamins and other nutrients.

Today, we produce 147 million metric tons of wheat every day, and much of this wheat is processed into white flour. Why is this flour white? Well, all the outer nutrient-dense layers have been removed to create a very shelf-stable simple carbohydrate that is in pretty much everything we eat today. This simple carbohydrate is broken down into sugar the minute we consume it. Hello diabetes! Sadly, as so many of the nutrients have been removed food manufactures have to add B vitamins back into the flour to make it nutritionally valid. There is one thing that certainly stays in the flour though, and that is the Roundup sprayed on it right before harvest. If that does not wake you up, then you are reading the wrong book.

There is more corn grown in the United States than any other crop. This is because corn is cheap and very easy to use for big food manufacturers to manipulate as fillers in food. This is done to make the food more palatable and stimulating to the reward centers of our brain. Watch out for these ultra-processed byproducts of GMO corn when you are reading food labels: corn flour, caramel flavor, corn fructose, corn meal, corn oil, corn syrup, dextrin, dextrose, fructose, lactic acid, malt, maltodextrin, monosodium glutamate (MSG), sorbitol, and most commonly, high fructose corn syrup. All of these are mass produced, unnatural and foreign to our body. They contain none of corn's nutritional benefits that an organic local corn kernel would because they are ultra-processed down to the simplest form to stimulate our brain's addiction to them.

High fructose corn syrup is a much cheaper way for big food to sweeten their chemically ridden lab-made "not food." This of course comes from GMO corn. As if sugar being added to everything to stimulate our brain is not bad enough, big food manufacturers now use a much cheaper form of sugar called fructose that comes from corn. One major problem with fructose is that it can only be metabolized in the liver, unlike glucose, which is the sugar molecule in cane sugar. The liver is a very big part of the detoxification of our body. The liver also plays a huge role in our blood sugar regulation, However, when it is loaded with high amounts of fructose, the liver can become overburdened and not able to properly detoxify the body, not to mention handle the blood sugar regulation. This causes an increase of toxins in our body as well as improperly regulated blood sugar, leading to a cascade of potential dis-ease.

The ultra-processing of vegetable oils makes them extremely toxic to our body. The majority of the oil is being processed from GMOs. They are not even close to an oil from a vegetable. Canola oil is one of the primary vegetable oils, and its name comes from the combination of Canadian oil, low acid. Canola oil is made from the ultra-processing of the rapeseed which was widely found in Canada. Other popular vegetable oils such as Crisco, Mazzola and Wesson are all primarily soybean oil mixed with about 15% corn, Canola, or peanut oil.

Oils are what are known chemically as lipids or fats. In food, fats (oils), enhance the flavor. They make foods more satiating by stimulating a fuller, richer taste. The food industry knows this, and they only have one motive—get you to buy their product so they can make more money. In order to do that, they need you to really, really love the taste of it. So, they have hired very smart biochemists to concoct a seemingly irresistible combination of carbohydrates (sugar), fat (oil) and protein, adding in all sorts of other flavors to stimulate the taste receptors in our brain. To lower their overall cost, they use the cheapest most satiating oils in these "not food" combinations.

Think of what it would take for you to squeeze oil out of a kernel of corn or a soy bean. A lot of pressure and heat. This is not an easy process, so in order to maximize production, toxic solvents are used. These further increase the inflammatory nature of such oils. The high heat used to process the oil from the plant causes the oil to be very unstable. Unstable means unbalanced. Now the body uses an oxidation-reduction process to try and balance out the chemical nature of these polyunsaturated fatty acids. This oxidation-reduction process causes inflammation all over the body as these lipids enter the blood stream.

Despite their load of toxins, such oils are cheap and provide a high surplus. Big food companies cannot resist. Nor can we as this oil is the backbone of the perfect taste combination that makes those Doritos impossible to put down. The majority of the ultra-processed bagged, packaged, boxed and canned food found in your grocery store comes from just a few plants processed cheaply into a food-like substance our body does not recognize. Bread, crackers, cookies, cereal, chips, soups, salad dressings, meat, etc. all have these crops in them in some way, shape or form.

Stay away from these toxic polyunsaturated fatty acid oils: canola, corn, cottonseed, peanut, safflower, sunflower, soybean and all other vegetable oils.

246

## Problem # 3—GMOs and Agrochemicals

Glyphosate is the active ingredient found in Roundup and is the most widely used herbicide in the world. Roundup is the brand name of a systemic, broad spectrum herbicide that was originally produced by Monsanto, but was bought by Bayer in 2018. It is Monsanto's, now Bayer's, star product among all agrochemicals.

The WHO (World Health Organization) has classified glyphosate as "probably carcinogenic in humans" in May 2015. In that same investigation, the WHO also found that glyphosate is probably genotoxic (which means it causes mutations in DNA). They found that it also increases oxidative stress, which causes inflammation in the body.

Of course, Monsanto claimed the WHO did not properly conduct the study and ignored dozens of other conflicting studies that showed glyphosate to be safe and non-toxic. However, it was later discovered that all the studies, which Monsanto claimed showed glyphosate to be nontoxic, were either funded by Monsanto or a different agrochemical company.[9]

Roundup and glyphosate are obviously not naturally occurring. And there is obviously something going on with our overall health in America. When we mix the disease-causing effects of living in chronic stress with the disease-causing effects of genetically altered food heavily sprayed with agrochemicals, it is not hard to connect the dots. Just think about the toxic foods we eat seeping through our leaky gut and into our blood stream. This alters our genetic program by turning on pro-inflammatory genes leading to a downhill cascade of possible diseases. These ultra-processed chemically altered "not foods" are signaling the genes of disease through epigenetics. The cell receives the signal and turns on the gene to create more inflammation to do something about this unknown foreign chemical, food particle or antibiotic in the system. Whether it is in the mouth, the gut or in our blood after it has leaked through the intestinal wall lining, the message is clear; this is foreign, and in consequence, inflammatory genes are turned on.

Why doesn't everybody experience allergies or symptoms from these foods? Quite simply, we are all unique. This is the same reason why one diet does not work for everyone. We all have a nearly infinite cascade of genes being switched on or switched off every millisecond. And dependence on where our stress level is at a conscious and subconscious level sets the stage. Factors like use of antibiotics previously in our life, current medications, cleanliness of local water, air pollution, mold toxicity and many other variables play into how each person will tolerate the toxic load of the conventional food we are all subject too.

It is not that corn, wheat and soy are inherently bad. They are not. The issue is that they are overgrown on a massive scale, ultra-processed to excite our palate and manipulated by genetically modified organisms all geared toward the profit of a powerful few companies.

So, what do we do? How do we make a change?

## Does Organic Really Matter?

Yes, it most definitely does. Again, we have to come back to awareness. Knowing what we are eating, where it comes from, whether we have good vibes from the manufacturer and how we have felt in the past when eating it all come into play. Buying organic vegetables is not always easy financially, and it is almost impossible to eat organic all the time because of the drastic shift in our agricultural practices. Many feel that organic is a marketing technique so companies can charge more for their product. No doubt it is used to market the product, but we also must consider the marketing manipulation that has been going on in the big food industry since we were kids eating Lucky Charms. The package coloring, food commercials catering to our cravings, product placement on grocery store shelves, bakery smells in grocery stores, sale prices, brand name recognition, and many other tactics are all marketing techniques.

The truth is, if you buy organic, you are giving your body a better chance not to have to deal with the toxic load of GMO and agrochemicals. Organic means, no GMO and no Roundup or any other chemical sprayed on the crop. This is giving your body a chance to heal and not to turn on so many inflammatory genes. Yes, you might have to pay a little more for an organic product, but consider the cost of your health. Can you put a price tag on it?

The same thing goes for organically raised animals. If the animal is organic, it is given no GMO feed, and no grasses it is grazing on are sprayed with Roundup. We will discuss properly raised healthy animals in a few pages.

An easier way to eat organic food and save the world is buying from local organic farmers. By buying their products, you are supporting a local company you believe in, giving back to earth its resources, and eating authentic, whole organic food, giving your body more nutrients to be put to good use. Our focus should be buying from local organic regenerative farmers more so than Whole Foods as it is the most powerful thing we can do to create change. When we buy from local organic farmers, we are doing our part to reduce the amount of carbon dioxide being used for these huge grocers to distribute their groceries from processing plant to store.

Back to marketing, many organic health food companies have been bought up by the big nine. Remember, they are all mainly concerned with the bottom line. Sell, sell, sell. So organic sugar added to all the organic chips, crackers, cereals, breads, and pastas is just as dangerous to your chance of becoming pre-diabetic as regular sugar. Same thing goes for organic sunflower, safflower, soybean and canola oil. We must be aware of a huge market for "health food," but just because it is marketed as healthy does not mean it is.

## What NOT to Eat?

In this section we shall consider food stuffs that you should try to avoid. Some are insidious in the sense that you find them in many products where you would not expect to see them. Only by becoming a conscientious and attentive label reader can you avoid such pitfalls.

### *Gluten*

Eliminate gluten. Gluten is a protein found in wheat.[10] Alessio Fasano has found gluten to trigger the unlocking of the epithelial cell lining of the intestinal tract. Remember that the lining of the gut is only one cell thick, and when there is space between or leaks, it enables toxic chemicals, undigested food particles and a whole host of other things meant to stay out of our blood to leak into it. This does not only happen in the individuals who have the celiac gene either. This happens in everyone's gut.

When gluten is digested and broken into its smaller parts, there are opioid chemicals in it called gluteomorphins that seep into the blood stream as well. These opioids trigger the same receptors in your brain that drugs like heroin do. This is why bread is extremely addictive. I remember when I decided to eliminate gluten from my diet, going through a period when I actually panicked at the thought of not having bread with a meal. I could not imagine not having some sort of gluten containing substance with a meal. The panic then turned into a bit of anger. Guided by Dave Asprey,

I had a plan of action about what I was going to eat, but looking back on that moment, I now understand I was going through withdrawal.

With the knowledge and understanding of this component of eliminating gluten from your diet, you will better understand what your body is going through when it is having a temper tantrum like a 5-year-old child who does not get a toy he or she wants.

Is it Gluten or is it Glyphosate?

Remember wheat is heavily sprayed with RoundUp right before harvest, begging the question whether it is the gluten bothering me or the RoundUp? They do not use this practice in most European wheat harvesting, and there are numerous stories of folks who have gluten intolerance traveling to Europe, enjoying an Italian pasta dish or pizza, and experiencing none of the symptoms they would have in the United States. As I have healed and sealed my gut wall lining, I have enjoyed a piece of organic sourdough bread or organic Italian dough pizza and have felt absolutely fine.

To understand your body and learn more about yourself, however, you should eliminate gluten to cool and calm the inflammatory load of the gut. Eliminate for 21 days to give your body a proper chance to heal and seal. The epithelial cells in your gut are constantly regenerating and renewing. By combining the elimination of gluten, sugar, corn, soy and conventional dairy, you will give your body a full cellular reset.

Then you can slowly start to introduce small amounts of organic wheat back into your diet. As you introduce this back in, make sure you know if the wheat is organic so you have a better understanding of whether it is the wheat or the glyphosate. You must also be conscious of the ingredients of the bread, cracker, etc. to weed out any other triggers. You know best.

**Sugar** (high-fructose corn syrup, honey, coconut sugar, brown sugar, maple syrup, brown rice syrup, sucrose, sucralose, aspartame)

Dopamine is a neurochemical that is released in our brain when we like something. Whether its sugar, sex, praise, alcohol, drugs, etc., dopamine is released, telling our brain and body we got a reward. Dopamine's purpose is for our survival. When it comes to food and survival, the release of dopamine when we eat something sweet was a very necessary survival technique. Quite simply, sweet equals more energy for the body to use in order to survive. More energy equals a better chance of survival. As for the sweetness of fruit which comes from the sugar fructose, this ensures we will not only have energy but store fat in our body for the winter months when food is not so readily available. Fat is stored to be utilized for energy at a later time. Another survival technique. Remember fructose skips a step of glycolysis and goes right to the liver to be metabolized, causing more fat to be stored. Either way, the brain absolutely loves sweet. It craves it, it remembers where it got it, and it has a hard time with portion control of it. This is all primarily because of the release of dopamine. Understanding that this is a primitive survival mechanism built in you will help eliminate sugar from your diet.

This knowledge also gives you some insight into why sugar or high fructose corn syrup is in nearly everything made by food companies. It is clearly obvious it triggers the center in your brain to make you want more. If you want more, you buy more, and they make more money. To me, this is almost criminal since the trickle-down effects on our health ultimately contribute to death. Tell me why in God's beautiful green earth does sugar need to be added to fruit products like canned fruit, fruit juice or jam? Sugar in ketchup, cold cuts, relish, peanut butter, mayonnaise, salad dressing, canned soup, cottage cheese, bread and pickles? Seriously? If you cannot see through the veil of what big food companies are doing to us to trick us to buy their product, then, again, you are reading the wrong book.

In order to cut the cord, to quit the habit, you have to quit eating it. Period.

## Processed Corn Product

GMO corn is in pretty much all things in a box or a bag you can find at the grocery store. As you have learned, GMO corn epigenetically turns on inflammatory disease-causing genes. The body does not recognize this as food, and by eliminating it, you are furthering your chance to heal and regenerate. In packaged, ultra-processed not food, the high carbohydrate GMO corn byproducts are almost always mixed with highly toxic refined oils. This creates the irresistible satiating product being sold. As for our health, this is a double-edged sword of inflammation in your body. The blood sugar spike of the carbohydrate from the corn or wheat mixed with the highly unstable vegetable oil causes many problems in the arteries of your blood vessels.

## Soy

Soy has a very strong effect on the hormone estrogen. It contains a component that binds to the same receptors of a cell that estrogen does. Now estrogen cannot signal the cell like it normally would as the soy molecule is taking up its loading and landing docks. Epigenetically this causes the cell to create a different protein than it normally would. This can cause problems systemically. However, this systemic disruption is widely determined by the overall health of the individual. In other words, how well balanced their hormonal function is. Again, the processing of soy into its byproducts of protein and oil are not recognized by the body and can have a disease-causing effect. This, in conjunction with the hormone mismanagement created by chronic stress, is another double-edged sword.

## Conventionally Raised Dairy

Just as toxins from industrialized farming can end up in the animals' meat, it also ends up in the animals' milk. As you know, these chemical toxins signal inflammatory genes in our body. The dairy industry is very large, and these industrial farmed cows are being manipulated by man to produce more milk than their bodies are intended to. This is done by adding hormones to their body to trick it into thinking it needs to continue producing milk. Again, this is a tactic used for increased profit.

The dairy cows of today have been bred to have a high level of a protein called A1 casein in their milk. Because the way A1 casein signals the genes of our body, it is a much more inflammatory protein to our body compared to A2 casein. A2 casein was present in the cows of yesteryear. A1 casein also produces another inflammatory and addictive peptide called casomorphin. There is that morphine again, just like the protein gluten has a downstream effect of gluteomorphin. And you guessed it—it is highly addictive. It also triggers the same part of the brain that addictive drugs signal. Think how many people absolutely love cheese. Have you seen the cheese section at the grocery store?

All store-bought milk goes through a pasteurization process. This is essentially a heating process where the cow's milk gets baked to a certain temperature to kill potentially harmful bacteria like E. coli, Listeria and Salmonella. The only problem is it also kills all the other beneficial bacteria in the milk that help our bodies as well as the calves break down the milk parts like casein to better digest them. It also goes through another process called homogenization. This is when the milk is squeezed through a tiny metal shaft at a high heat temperature to "flatten" its particles and make the milk a consistent color, giving it uniformity. The problem is this high-pressured squeezing changes the shape of the milk fats, fatty acid tails. In macro, the fats behave by the way they are shaped, and these misshapen fatty acids can be detected as a foreign object after ingesting.

Because we have been misguided that fat is bad, low-fat milk has been created. By removing the fat from the milk, we have taken essential and life-sustaining fat from the milk and created a very consistent, white, sugary (lactose), shelf-stable drink that everyone "should" be drinking in order to get the calcium they need for "strong bones." This is what we were told, and we believe it. But this is just another marketing technique, driven by the dairy industry. There are plenty of other beneficial ways to get the calcium we need in our diet. Here again, this white, consistent drink is not milk, it is a manmade substance that has been over-processed, taking it very far away from its God-given intent.

An aside on the bacteria we have been told are so bad and will make us sick and kill us. We now live in an antibacterial world. Antibiotics given for every ailment by the doctor, anti-bacterial soap, anti-bacterial hand sanitizers everywhere, anti, anti, anti! When using these chemical toxic products, we are killing all the tiny living organisms that have been here way longer than us. We live in symbiosis with trillions of bacteria, fungi and viruses during every second of our day. Do you not think there is a reason for that? Yet, we are told these germs will make us sick, and they are bad! We need to scrub ourselves with "certain" products that will kill them and keep us safe. It has gone too far. I mean I am all for being clean, I love how I feel after a shower. But it is obvious to me the fear created by the potential sickness these deemed "bad" germs can create is a total marketing ploy playing into the narrative that pharmaceutical drugs are the fix rather than looking to our innate capacity.

An interesting theory I think should be given some thought and more study is that these bacteria are there to naturally decompose the toxicity of our modern world. For example, take listeria found in milk. Perhaps the cow has been exposed to a toxic environment, eating GMO feed heavily sprayed with RoundUp, and the listeria is in her milk as a byproduct of nature trying to clean her body of the toxic world she's living in. Now her milk is ingested by a human, and they get sick. We test the milk, and we find listeria. Now this is where the question arises of how do we know it was the listeria that made the human sick? Well, to the best of my knowledge and Thomas Cowan's (which is where I learned this), in order to isolate this hypothesis, we would need to use what are called the Koch postulates. Koch postulates were created by the German physician named Robert Koch in 1890, and they are used to determine whether a given bacteria or virus is the cause of a given disease. There are four criteria that make common sense.

1. The bacteria must be present in every case of the disease.

    a. In the case of listeria in milk, everyone who drank the milk and got sick would need to test positive for listeria.

2. The bacteria must be isolated from the host and grown in pure culture.

3. The disease must be reproduced when the pure culture of the bacteria is inoculated into a healthy susceptible host.

4. The bacteria must be recoverable from the experimentally infected host.

If each one of those four postulates are proven, then we can say it was, in fact, the listeria in the milk. However, I would argue that this deductive reasoning is rarely ever done. So how do we know if it was the bacteria found in the milk or the toxic chemical found in the milk that made the host puke their guts out? We do not. But the listeria gets blamed because there is a profitable medicine to kill it classified as an antibiotic. End aside.

## Toxic Vegetable Oil

Eating plenty of healthy fat is a cornerstone of regaining health in your life as you will see in a few paragraphs. Nevertheless, to a large degree, the toxic ultra-processed vegetable oils we learned about before have replaced the natural whole fat in our diet. Big food companies love refined polyunsaturated oils like corn, canola, sunflower and safflower because they are cheap to manufacture, easy to transport and do not spoil easily, giving them an extra-long shelf life. Consumers love these toxic oils as they are rewarding to our taste buds. This sounds wonderful until we examine what they are doing to our health, however, big food companies are still trying to blame butter and coconut oil. While their artificially extracted oils go through the high heat processing called hydrogenation. As we talked about before, think of what it takes to squeeze oil out of a kernel of corn or a soybean not to mention the solvents needed to expedite this process. This processing makes the oil very rancid as it creates a highly reactive lipid that is very unstable because of its chemical structure. As this fatty acid gets digested and enters our blood, it needs to become more stable by attracting or stealing an electron. Because of the very massive amounts of poly-unsaturated fatty acids (PUFA) found in modern vegetable oils, we do not have enough antioxidants such as Vitamin E to account for or balance these unstable PUFAs causing an inflammatory storm. As you start to read the labels of grocery store food boxes, bags and packages, you see these oils everywhere. The scale is tipped to these inflammatory oils, and if we eat the Standard American Diet, it is simply too much for our bodies to handle, causing an inflammation explosion leading to dis-ease in the body.

I want to reiterate the fact that inherently corn, wheat, soy and sugar are not bad. Do not worry! This does not mean you can never eat these foods again. You can when they are in whole organic form, but first you must allow your body to heal through the elimination of them.

## What to Eat

The simple, but very important message in this section is that you should eat loads of the highest quality vegetables you can find.

Vegetables should become what we base our meals around. This is difficult, I know, as animal protein is usually the foundational piece of our meal. However, eating more vegetables will catapult your body's healing process. As you know, the health of the soil is vital to our health, so when we eat fresh organic vegetables, we are receiving the bounty of nutrients absorbed into the plant from the earth. Quality of the vegetables definitely matters, as it should be grown in the most organically diverse soil you know of. However, in today's store-bought world, it is hard to know how healthy the soil is from which the broccoli you just bought came from.

So do your best to buy organic products you believe in and have done some research on. But again remember, the best way to become educated on your food is to buy your produce from a local farmer's market. This is a great way to learn about the soil and the farming practices of the local produce you are purchasing. When produce is fresh, it carries more nutrient density. Especially compared to when it is flown in on 747 jets from across the globe and sits in plastic packaging. The food's nutrient potency is lost, and air pollution is gained. Buying from your local organic farmer's market ensures that the produce is closer to its peak of nutrient benefit. This is also very beneficial for the earth as you are supporting farmers that are restoring the microbiome of the soil. Your money goes straight to the farmer, supporting their hard work and efficacy. Your dollar is probably the most powerful way for you to make an impactful change to save our earth. This is a win, win, win, for you, the farmer and the earth.

Furthermore, the plants themselves are alchemists and create magic within their roots, stems flowers and, in turn, within us. Powerful immune boosting antioxidants and phytochemicals come packaged in both micro and macronutrient components to assist our body in maintaining health and vitality. Through their amazing chemistry, the edible plant kingdom has manufactured medicine for the symbiotic relationship of plant, animal, earth (soil), water and air. On the most fundamental level it is so obvious that we should love and cherish the plant kingdom for the simple fact that we must have their oxygen to breathe, and they must have our carbon dioxide to breathe. We use what they exhale, and they use what we exhale. Talk about the circle of life. To me it is a no-brainer that the earth and its plants should be at the top of our priority list.

These plants manufacture phytochemical components that create the following in our body:

- Antioxidation: flavonoids found in fruits and vegetables oxidize free radicals, helping our body's tissues from breaking down.

- Stimulation of enzymes: indoles found in cabbage help to stimulate enzymatic operation, creating proper cell function to manufacture and create life giving proteins.

- Interference with DNA replication: capsaicin found in red peppers, protects DNA from carcinogens, thereby preventing cancer replication.

- Physical actions: cranberries have a phytochemical called proanthocyanidins which binds to the cell wall, creating an anti-adhesion blockage of pathogens that can cause urinary tract infections as well as prevention of pathogens binding to teeth and gums in the mouth.

These are a very few examples of the medicine found in plants.

So why would we not want to increase our consumption of a diverse number of vegetables? Well, this is again, where education creates awareness. If we know the magic of the plant kingdom is medicine, we will likely want to eat more plants and vegetables. When we understand that the SAD has hijacked our reward system in our brain, creating an addiction to sweet and palatable not foods, we have a better foundation to make a conscious choice not to eat what we know is disease-causing in our body. This is the first step. The second step is to have some knowledge of how to make vegetables taste good.

We are going to quite literally butter them up. As we discussed earlier, fat (oil) creates a flavor effect in food. It makes the food tastier. This is why toxic oils are added to almost all the ultra-processed foods in the grocery store. Well, we will learn in the paragraphs to come that there are healthy fats and why these should be an absolute staple in a healthy diet. One of the best of the healthy fats is butter that comes from a grass-fed only cow. And when you melt butter on hot steamed vegetables topped with sea salt, you have an amazing, tasty health food. Erase the belief that was instilled in you via marketing that fat is bad and load up your veggies with grass-fed butter. Another way to start loving vegetables is to roast them in the oven with avocado oil, olive oil or ghee. I like to chop up cauliflower, cabbage, red onion, carrots, squash and mushrooms, throw it all into a big bowl and coat with avocado oil, then spread out on a rimmed cookie sheet and bake in the oven at 350° for about 20-25 minutes, less or more to your likening. The baking brings out amazing flavors, which combined with a healthy fat, allows for all fat-soluble vitamins to be properly absorbed.

**An aside** Ghee is clarified butter, which is butter that has been melted in order to remove the milk solids. This leaves only the fat or oil of the butter. The milk solids are what contain lactose, caseins, whey proteins and minerals from the milk. This leaves a stable cooking oil for higher temperatures so the proteins and sugars do not burn, allowing just the fatty acids, which stay intact. Each oil has a smoke point that has been determined. When the oil or fat is heated past its smoke point, the oil will start to denature and release free radicals in your food. We want to avoid free radicals as they are what break down tissues in our body. Antioxidants are free radical scavengers, chemically bonding with them to decrease their inflammatory nature. Butter has a smoke point of 350° while ghee has a smoke point of 485°. Coconut oil's smoke point is 350°, and refined avocado oil has a smoke point of 500° while unrefined virgin avocado oil's smoke point is 350-375°. We will cover the processing of healthy oils in the adding healthy fat section below.

In general, the vegetable to fruit ratio should be 80/20. 80% vegetables and 20% fruit. Healthy traditional peoples often ate a very large number and variety of vegetables. They included root vegetables like carrots, yams, yucca, and jicama. They added leafy green vegetables such as kale, broccoli, bok choy, collard greens, spinach and cabbage as well as fruit vegetables like squash, avocados, cucumbers, peppers, tomatoes and olives. The diversity of their diet compared to the SAD was massive. To me, it is just common sense that their health would benefit and ours is the worst it has ever been. Most Americans do not even know what bok choy is. I did not until I learned to love vegetables.

Just like any kind of change, your body is going to throw a fit about changing your diet. Go back to your intuition. There is a reason you wanted to change. You want to heal. You want to be in control of your life. You want to feel the love in you, making it greater and stronger every second. Your ego does not like change. It wants instant gratification. Then it wants to make you feel guilty for it. This is not who you really are. These are low-energy emotions to give you a fix and to manipulate you into irrational decisions. You now are greater than that because you have raised your consciousness.

## Protein. Animal or Plant

It is not my intent to persuade you to eat animal meat or not eat it, but it is my intent to share with you the importance of protein. In Greek, protein means primary. That is number one. We now understand that when we talk about proteins, we are talking about the structure and the function of the body. And we know the genes in all our cells (over a trillion of them) in the body produce proteins that go off and do a specific job. They replenish our muscle cells, our bones, ligaments, and joints. They help the function of our eyes, our brain, our heart, our liver, etc. They replenish and regenerate our skin, hair and nails. Everything and everywhere in our body. Inside the cell, the DNA and RNA must have the proper amino acid building blocks in order for them to manufacture new healthy proteins. Amino acids are what proteins are made of. It makes sense, then, that if we feed our body the healthiest proteins we can find, we will have the healthiest building blocks of amino acids to transcribe new proteins. When we give our body this nourishing protein, it then can break the food down into the essential amino acids our DNA and RNA need to transcribe and manufacture new proteins. Now these new and vibrant, healthy proteins go on to create new and vibrant structures and functions within every cell of our body. We now know how important our gut is for the proper breakdown of the proteins, and we also know how to improve its function.

It does not make sense that our body can achieve maximum health and vitality by eating sick plants or animals. When it comes to choosing our protein, this makes our decision process pretty simple on what to buy. Did this animal live a healthy and happy life? What would be the most natural habitat for this animal or plant to thrive? If the animal is healthy and happy, then that is what we are eating. Same questions go for plant protein.

## Animal Protein. Grass-Fed, Pastured or Wild

Cows are meant to eat grass, that is it. However, because of profit, we have found they become fatter (remember fat is more satiating) and can go to market quicker when we feed them corn, soy and hay (alfalfa). If the farmer is pumping out acres and acres of GMO corn, soy and alfalfa and being subsidized to do so, it would make sense that those crops could not only be processed into our Doritos but also feed our ribeye steaks we raked in from the grocery store for $5 a pound. Much of our corn, wheat, alfalfa and soy production is used for cattle feed in the US. This makes the industrialized meat much cheaper by speeding up the target weight for an animal to reach since the animal fattens quickly from eating these crops.

$5 a pound for a ribeye! What? Where? Without even asking what the animal ate or if it was humanely raised, we jump to get the deal. We are obsessed with saving money at the grocery store, just as the grocery store is obsessed with making money off marking things up. But where is this food coming from and why is ground beef so readily available and cheap? We must wake up to what is going on and the massive implications the aforementioned process has on our health and the health of our planet.

As cows are only meant to eat grass, when they eat corn, grains and hay, their stomachs do not take all that well to it. As this improper feeding occurs throughout their lives, the cows' immune system is weakened because their digestive system is compromised and inflamed. Being immunocompromised, they are now more susceptible to disease. Not to mention, industrially farmed cattle are not living in a healthy way, packed into feedlots like sardines and wading in their own and all the other cattle's excrement. The end result is they get sick. In an effort to keep these cattle from dying (because that is not profitable), the cheaper alternative is to routinely give these cattle broad-spectrum anti-biotics. Anti-biotics kill all bacteria, good and bad. The pathogens meant to be killed become resistant to overused broad-spectrum antibiotics and are able to over-grow causing an even greater imbalance. These anti-biotics are not only excreted through the cattle's waste, but they are in the tissue we eat. And their potency is affecting our gut microbiome as well, furthering our microbiota imbalance.

We have to question what is in our food and what our food is eating. As Steven Gundry says, you are not just what you eat, you are what you eat, ate. In other words, if an animal is fed nutrient-depleted, chemically altered, toxic food, then we are eating that same thing when we eat the animal meat or ingest their milk products.

Chickens are omnivores that are meant to forage for food, scratching and picking the earth for insects as well as plants, vegetables and fruit when available. Today, chickens are fed the cheapest combination of corn, soy and other grains. Same thing goes with chicken, what they eat is what we eat. How about the chickens' eggs? If the chicken is fed a manmade concoction to increase their growth as quickly as possible, then that is what we are ingesting in our conventional eggs as well. Have you ever seen a bright golden yolk of a pasture-raised chicken compared to a conventionally raised chicken that produces the $2 a dozen eggs? If you have not, you should look up a picture of it on the Internet. Just search pastured egg yolk compared to conventional. The more golden and bright the yolk, the healthier the chicken. Then there is the anti-biotics and growth hormones being pumped into these poor things. Again, if it is being put into them, it is being put into us.

Salmon has been called one of nature's most perfect foods. For it has a beautiful combination of nutrition our body can use and assimilate the way it should. To increase production and profit, however, salmon fish farms have become more prevalent. Here again, large amounts of fish are living in an unnatural environment and fed a manmade concoction of GMO soy and conventional grains. This causes the fish to be nutrient devoid as compared to wild caught salmon. Also, like the concentrated animal feeding operations mentioned above, thousands of these fish are crammed into pens that leads to parasite growth and diseases, which heavy use of anti-biotics and pesticides are used to prevent.

If you eat pork, make sure the pigs are living in an environment where they have time to dig in the forest with their snouts. You should also make sure the pig is fed organic feed. And a lamb is meant to be on pasture and eat grass, clover, forbs and whatever else grows in an organic pasture.

The same way your body will thrive and flourish when you take off all the masks you have been wearing and become who you truly are, these animals need to be who they are as well, living, eating and playing in the way most compatible with their true nature. Think about it. By allowing these animals to be who and what they are, we are not only respecting them as living and vital creatures of this earth, but we are creating harmony and health in their bodies. This makes for the sacrifice of these animals to be much more sustainable to their species and our planet. We can truly honor their lives and the nourishment they provide for our bodies as prayer before a meal was intended.

As protein has become the main course of our meals, the portion size has consequently increased. This has played into the factory farming of animals yielding high profits for manufactures. More, more, more. With money and profit driving the industrialization of animals for our increasing demands, the animal has been looked at as lower and separate from the human species. Over the years, this has led to a monopoly of the entire food industry from agriculture to agrochemicals to cattle feedlots to chicken industry to pork, all in the name of a bigger, cheaper per pound, more marbled with fat ribeye. It has led to corrupt science, which is not even science, just manipulation. It has even led to shipping animals overseas to be slaughtered and then sent back to America. When you step back and look at it from a different perspective, it seems disgusting and even criminal.

My point is that we do not need as much protein as our greedy bellies tell us we do. We should only be eating about the portion size of our fist or a deck of cards in one day. If we are very active and athletic, we should probably double that in a day. There is some fantastic science out there showing the dangers of eating too much protein. Valter Longo has pointed out the disease-causing effects of eating too much animal protein.

This brings us to plant proteins. Plants have proteins in them and certain plants have more than others. There is much debate about which is better, plant or animal protein, however, there is no point in arguing between the two. The point here is to educate you on what to eat to get these essential proteins from plants no matter whether you choose to go vegan, paleo, ketogenic or a combination of the three.

Scientists have found 21 amino acids that, in different combinations, make up all the proteins in our body. Nine of these 21 considered essential can only be obtained from food. Animal proteins like grass-fed beef, pasture-raised chicken and turkey, wild-caught fish, grass-fed organic dairy and pasture-raised eggs contain plenty of each of the nine essential amino acids, thus, they are considered complete proteins. Plants on the other hand do not have as bountiful amounts of the essential amino acids or are missing some of the nine but do have higher amounts of the others. Eating a wide variety of plant protein covers all the bases. And as we have learned, eating a diverse number of plants is great for your health.

Here is a list of some good sources of plant proteins: Tempeh (fermented soy, grain free only), Hillary's Root veggie burger (root veggies mixed with millet), Quorn (brand name) Hemp tofu, Hemp seeds, Millet, organic sprouted beans, amaranth, nutritional yeast, chia seeds, spirulina, quinoa, nuts (almonds, walnuts, macadamia, pistachios, Brazil nuts, coconut, pine nuts, flaxseeds, sesame seeds, chestnuts).

## *Good Fats*

Eating good amounts of healthy fat is essential for your health. Every cell in your body is lined with a phospholipid bilayer, which is made entirely of fat. Remember when we learned about the cell's memBRAIN? Well, this is made from fat. All cells receive and give information through the cell membrane and a healthy phospholipid bilayer will only improve our cellular function. This means healthy fat must be a staple in our diet.

It is very unfortunate that we have been told fat makes you fat. In the late 1980s recommendations were made to start eliminating fat from our diets. A transition has since ensued of using ultra-processed vegetable oils, and we have just gotten sicker and fatter ever since. These have been marketed as cholesterol free and healthy, however, the chronic disease influx tells us something is not right.

Aside from fat lining every cell in our body, being the conduit to direct cellular messages from cell to cell, fats also make up a large portion of our brain matter. Merely because our brain is made of around 60% fat, we must replenish these building blocks of lipids by eating a higher percentage of healthy fats in our diet to be utilized for neuroplasticity and regeneration in our brain. Remember how we talked about neurodegenerative diseases being a problem of the demyelination of nerve cells? Well, myelin is a fatty tissue that lines the axon of the nerve cell. It is made up of about 70% saturated fat and cholesterol (which is a fat—both of which we have been told are bad for us). In order to create myelin synthesis in our brain to replenish our neurons, we NEED cholesterol in order for this biochemical process to take place.

As we will learn in more detail during the intermittent fasting section, when we do not eat carbohydrates for a certain period, our body starts to use its own fat reserves for fuel. By adding healthy fat into our diet during this time of carbohydrate restriction, we can help train our metabolism to use fat for energy. This is a great way to decrease inflammation in the entire body and feed the brain powerful fats to optimize its function, giving us more focus and mental clarity since there are no sugar spikes to disrupt cellular homeostasis. Remember that fat is a carrier of flavor as it upregulates the taste receptors from our tongue to our brain? In a similar fashion, its chemical components are satiating as well. This means that eating fat makes us less hungry. As you know with sweets and the combination of sweet and salty, we can continue to eat while not being satisfied.

When we teach our body's metabolism to use and break down fat for fuel, we become satisfied and energized without feeling the crash of carbohydrates after the blood sugar spike they create. This can include protein too. An example of a high-fat meal with protein and no carbohydrates would be eggs cooked in butter or avocado oil and sautéed asparagus in either oil as well. Another example is an omelet with spinach, mushrooms, onions and served with an avocado on top. Eliminating the carbohydrate while adding healthy fat and even protein can be a gateway to a cleaner burning, less inflammatory body.

## Good Fats. Reducing Calcification

Vitamins A, D, E and K are all fat-soluble vitamins, and they are abundant in many of the recommended foods in this section. This means for these vitamins to be absorbed into our system, they need fat. These vitamins are essential in the proper placement of calcium into our bones and teeth. Calcium is essential for numerous functions in the body. It is the most abundant mineral in the body, and its placement being in the right tissues, like bone and teeth, and not being too high in the bloodstream is essential for our health.

When we eat a diet high in carbohydrates (i.e. the SAD), it causes calcium, B vitamins, magnesium and other minerals to be taken from bone and teeth and be used for other enzyme processes needed to deal with the elevated glucose in the blood. Because of the overabundance of sugar in the blood, our body releases the base-forming minerals like calcium and magnesium from our bone to balance the blood pH. In other words, because of the high amounts of sugar in the SAD, we are robbing our bones of this precious mineral calcium. This is the body's way of keeping homeostasis, but unfortunately, prolonged eating this way can cause things like tooth decay, osteopenia, osteoporosis, susceptibility to fractures, kidney stones, tendon injuries, arthritis, etc.

Not only is it robbing our bones and teeth of this precious mineral, it causes the calcium level in the blood to be too high. With an overabundance of calcium in the blood, the calcium ion connects to our organs and the tissues in our body. This is because the blood goes everywhere. Over time, the calcium starts to cause problems like hardening of the tissue. Remember calcium is used to make bone, so in a sense it is developing hard bone-like disruptors on and in the tissues and organs. This overabundance of calcium can end up many places in the body—like arteries of the heart, Achilles' tendon or the pineal gland in the third ventricle of the brain.

So where do healthy fats come in? These healthy fats mentioned above are not only full of vitamins A and K, but when we eat them with a bountiful amount of vegetables, we are getting the entire complex of the vitamins we need to properly distribute calcium into our bones and teeth. Proper digestion of these vitamins allows for calcium to be absorbed into our bones and teeth, keeping them strong. This in combination with the elimination of sugar from our diet, we lower our blood sugar and stop the release of calcium from our bones coming into the blood. When we get back to nature and enjoy being outside in the sun, we stimulate vitamin D production in our body. This creates a nutritional formula to balance the pH in our blood and keep bones and teeth healthy and strong. At the same time, we allow our soft tissues in the body to heal and regenerate, creating a strong, supple and springy tissue throughout our entire body.

Eating more 100% grass-fed and grass-finished butter or ghee will provide you with a wonderful combination of vitamins A, D,

E and K, all packaged in the fat it needs to be absorbed. Ghee has always been a sacred and celebrated symbol of nourishment and healing in India. It has been used for centuries as a super food by delivering digestive and elimination aid, for energy, sexual vitality, skin and eye health, as a lubricant for the joints and for alkalizing the blood.

## Smart vs Poor Carbohydrates

We need carbohydrates. They are energy-producing fuel for our body, but we must teach our metabolism how to be flexible. Because of the carbohydrate-rich SAD, our blood sugar sky rockets after a meal. Take a look at breakfast, for example. We are told it is the most important meal of the day. Eat your cereal, breakfast bars, pancakes, fruit, bagels, toast and jam. All carbohydrates and sugar which create one massive sugar spike in our blood. It is estimated that a westerner eats 300 plus grams of carbohydrates per day.

So, what happens? We get a rush, we get going, and then two hours later we crash. Our bodies are now looking for that sugar (carbohydrate). One of the primary reasons for this urgent message to eat more sugar and carbohydrates is that the sugar and carbohydrates release serotonin in the brain. This hormone boosts our mood and makes us feel good. We love this mood boost, making sugar and carbohydrates even more addictive. The body sends messages to the brain asking, "Where's my sugar?" I need it, it is what I know. Now the brain has to figure out what to do since it realizes it has to wait until lunch to eat, so it gets hangry (hungry + angry). We get hangry because our ego (the conditioned cells of the body) want their sugar, and they are sending urgent messages to the brain to get it. When the brain is overloaded with these urgent messages through the vagus nerve, the body and brain become imbalanced. There is anxiety within our system. This can make us angry because we are unsettled. Just as an addict would become angry when he or she doesn't have drugs. We have conditioned our body this way through the SAD. This is what it knows, just as a dog gets conditioned by a bell to food. This is a stimulus and response. The question is can we become aware of this process and be greater than it?

Having knowledge of why this is happening is our antidote—that and knowing what to eat and when to eat it. It is our job to be the scientist of our own life and learn what works best for our body. Because we have such a large frontal lobe, this allows us to be aware that we are aware. This means we have a choice, and we can choose to be greater than these powerful food addictions.

Chronically high blood sugar is inflammatory, thus eating a SAD is inflammatory. There is no way around it. When you spill a soda and do not wipe it up thoroughly, its remnants on the counter are very sticky. Honey, maple syrup, marshmallows, you name it—it is all sticky. Glucose (sugar) in the blood is no different. It is sticky. The sticky nature of it causes the glucose in the blood to stick to proteins and fat molecules in both the blood and tissues. This is a process called glycation. And glycation produces a harmful inflammatory compound called advanced glycation end products (AGEs). High levels of AGEs have been linked to the development of many diseases. Diseases like diabetes, heart disease, kidney failure, and Alzheimer's, not to mention premature ageing. Ironic that their acronym is AGE?

### *Timing & Carbohydrates*

If you feel energy crashes and fatigue throughout the day try this. Do not eat carbohydrates for breakfast. In fact, do not eat breakfast, or at least hold off on it for as long as you can in a fasted state. (Details to come as to why in the intermittent fasting section.) When we wake up in the morning, the hormone cortisol (the stress hormone) is elevated in our body to get us going. As you remember, this hormone is responsible for the transition of energy to our brain, heart and muscles to prepare us for survival. Well, that's not its only use as our body uses it all the time for getting us ramped up and ready to go in a similar fashion. However, the chronic mismanagement of our emotions (i.e., living in stress) is where the problem lies because of the overabundance of cortisol in our system.

Upon waking, cortisol works to liberate stored sugars, amino acids and fatty acids from our body fat to use as fuel, as it is the chief catabolic hormone. This design is the genius innate capacity from our body to get us up and going to create an amazing day. The minute we consume a carbohydrate upon waking, whether it's orange juice or oatmeal, we now elevate another hormone in our body called insulin. Once insulin is present, it shuts down the fat cells from releasing these stored fatty acids from our body fat for use as our fuel. Not only that, but thanks to the insulin spike from the carbohydrate, our body is signaled to store the excess carbohydrate intake as fat. This starts the rollercoaster of hunger and cravings spikes throughout the rest of the day as our insulin levels go up and down.

As an athlete, I was taught to carb load before a high-intensity event, such as a workout, practice or a game. This theory seems to make sense as the carbohydrates turn to glucose in our body and then our cells can use this glucose for energy. Simple right? Well, if it were that simple, then we would not be the most obese nation in the world because we would just burn off all that sugar and more. I mean we probably have the most gym memberships sold in the world too, but that does not seem to help. What gives?

Unfortunately, it is not as simple as calories in, calories out. When we consume our sugar-rich pre-workout meal, shake or bar, the resulting sugar overload emits a signal to the body to store it as fat—thanks to the insulin spike, it is making us fatter. However, the marketing stays the same.

To become metabolically flexible, and as we learn to fast intermittently and cut out the excessive carbohydrates and sugar from our diet, our body learns to utilize what it already has. After it burns through the constituents of the previous meal and then the glycogen stores in the liver, fatty acids from the adipose tissue are released to be turned into fuel for energy. This is a biochemical process called gluconeogenesis that your body already knows. It takes about 12 or so hours of not eating to get into gluconeogenesis.

If we have been living on the SAD, our brain has been trained for using glucose (sugar) as its main source of energy. We will be shifting into a fat-burning state, which can be a challenge for a lot of people since the body is going to throw a fit. Some have called this experience the "carb flu" as the body and brain are going through a metabolic shift and the brain is not getting its regular spike of serotonin and dopamine from the sugar.

As you become metabolically flexible, you will notice you are no longer hangry after going several hours without eating. Your cravings for the carbohydrate-rich and sugary snacks disappear between meals. Your mind is clear. You notice you have sharper focus. And your energy levels are up and stable, not crashing and feeling tired.

So, if we need carbohydrates, when do we eat them? After a workout or during our last meal of the day. By eliminating carbohydrates and using your body's innate capacity to use up reserves and generate energy from fat, it is performance enhancing to replenish the carbohydrate stores in your body. Just as the SAD is dumping massive amounts of sugar into the body all day every day, we do not want to rely solely on gluconeogenesis for fuel. After the body has worked all day or exercised and used up all the stores of glycogen, the muscles will suck up the incoming carbohydrates from the meal afterwards. So instead of "carb loading," we are "carb refeeding."

Normally insulin is needed to be present outside of the cell on its membrane to unlock a gate to allow glucose to enter. However, once we are fat adapted and metabolically flexible, after exercise, the cells of the muscle tissue now take in the glucose from the blood without even needing insulin to do so. These post workout carbohydrates are less likely to be stored as fat and more likely to be used in the muscle tissue, increasing muscle mass. This increase of muscle mass now causes an increase of our overall metabolism, creating a buffer for calories in our diet.

Eat smart carbohydrates for dinner. If you have worked a long hard day, especially if you have been on your feet walking or doing some sort of physical labor, eat carbohydrates at the end of the day for dinner. Same principle implies as after exercise. You have gone through your glycogen stores by moving and standing all day and can replenish them with enjoying a smart carbohydrate for dinner. Exercise does not have to be something that requires spandex and a sweatband. Exercise can be a wide variety of activities. When I speak of eating carbs after exercise, think about your overall physical activity for the day.

Here is a list of foods that are smart carbohydrates.

Siete brand tortillas, Siete brand chips, Sweet Potato or yams, Green Plantains, Green Bananas, Cassava, Yuca, white rice, Jicama, Turnips, Taro roots, Rutabaga, Green Mango, Green Papaya, Millet Sorghum

All the above carbohydrates are called resistant starches. Resistant starches get their name because they are "resistant" to digestion in the small intestines. This keeps them intact and too big to be digested into the blood stream. Usually, being a starch, they would be digested and turned into sugar in the small intestines, but not so with resistant starches. They travel all the way to the colon or large intestine. Here they do wonderful health-promoting things. In the colon, the resistant starch acts more like a prebiotic than a starch. A prebiotic is something that our good gut microbiome in our colon feeds on. And when they feed on resistant starches, they produce a byproduct called Butyrate (Butyric acid). This molecule is a short-chain fatty acid and is able to enter the bloodstream. Butyrate is also very high in grass-fed butter and ghee, which is one of the reasons these two fats should be a staple in your diet. This SCFA is the main fuel source for our colonocytes, the cells that make up our gut lining. Unlike most other cells using glucose for energy, these little health-producing cells of ours use SCFAs for fuel. This could be one reason this study performed in 2013 revealed mice that ate resistant-starch rich foods showed a decrease in the number and size of lesions tied to colon cancer.[11]

The mice in the same study also showed a high amount of IL-10, a protein that is used in anti-inflammation. Decrease the inflammation in your gut, and you are decreasing the inflammation in your system. The anti-inflammatory effects an increased overall function of the colonocytes, allowing the tissue to heal and seal, keeping other inflammatory toxins from leaking into the bloodstream.

### Smart Carbohydrate: Fruit

The most important fruits to include in your diet are organic or wild berries such as blueberries, raspberries, blackberries, strawberries, cranberries, goji berries, acai berries. These fruits pack a powerful antioxidant punch, not to mention their amazing taste. It is a great idea to eat organic and wild berries as your carbohydrate refeed after a workout or for dessert after dinner.

When consuming fruits, do your best to eat the fruits in their peak season. This means when nature would naturally produce these fruits. For example, wild blueberries are naturally abundantly ripe in the months of July and August in the North Central and North-East parts of North America. This is when the fruit has the most nutrient density and the least number of proteins called lectins that plants use as a toxin to defend against insects.

As humans we were never meant to eat fruit year-round. Fruit naturally ripens in the summer and fall months. In many climates, when winter came, the natives had loaded up on fruit through the summer and fall. Eating the abundant available fruits naturally added on some body fat to prepare for the lack of food the winter months brought. It all makes sense because the sugar that sweetens fruit is called fructose—the same sugar processed from corn in high fructose corn syrup. Remember fructose is metabolized mainly in the liver to replenish our storage of glycogen there, and when we have plenty glycogen stores in the liver, this excess sugar gets stored right into fat. With the combination of having fruit at our fingertips year-round and believing it is a healthy alternative, mixed with the SAD, fruit packs on the pounds. There is just too much sugar, and fructose does not help the matter. Here again, there is absolutely nothing wrong with fruit, but being conscious of when to eat it is the name of the game.

One more problem with too much fructose, whether from fruit or high fructose corn syrup, is that fatty acids are a byproduct of its metabolism, and the overabundance of these fatty acids can lead to nonalcoholic fatty liver disease. The liver is the body's filter, it cleanses and clears the blood of toxic waste. In the toxic world we live in, the liver is drowned in detoxifying work. From the agrochemicals in the SAD to the pollution in the air, to the mold in our coffee, to the allergens from the air, the toxic effects of pharmaceutical prescriptions, etc. Our liver can get overburdened and not have enough time to regenerate and repair. Unfortunately, a heavy diet of fruit just adds to the toxic burden of the liver. Maybe you are asking, "Ok, but how do we give our liver a break to detoxify?" Great question! Intermittent fasting is your solution. Of course, that is mixed in with your daily dose of meditation!

## Intermittent Fasting

Intermittent fasting can be an absolute game changer to our health. It can catapult you into the best version of yourself in a matter of weeks by rewiring your cellular function right back into its homeostatic sweet spot, leaving you feeling like you again—having a crystal clear brain and vibrant healthy cells in the body.

Think about this, who does it benefit to buy all the "not food" and eat three square meals a day with snacks in between? Not to mention in each of those meals having some sort of grain being the staple (i.e. the old food pyramid). Furthermore, think about this. What happens to our blood sugar when these carbohydrate-heavy meals are eaten regularly throughout the day? It goes up every time we eat, right? Day in, day out, all day we are bombarding our cells with sugar. The body never gets a break from sugar. We eat it before bed (ice cream), and then we wake up and eat it first thing in the morning (cereal). The body is loaded with it. And you have learned why sugar cravings are so powerful.

The only reason we believe we need to eat breakfast is because it is what we have been sold. We were told the brain and body need breakfast for energy, so it is imperative we eat it. Otherwise, we will not be able to function. We learn this at a very early age in school, from our parents, from television, everywhere. We are programmed to eat breakfast because it makes us strong and healthy.

This is a story, and it could not be any further from the truth. Who made this story up? It was actually an ingenious marketing plan from Mr. Kellogg's Corn Flakes himself, the father of breakfast cereal. Needing to eat breakfast every day is an absolute fallacy. It is based on an outdated food pyramid that says carbohydrates should be the primary calorie load in the meal. Do not forget what you put on your breakfast cereal. Got milk? A double whammy of processed, high sugar "not food." This old story of breakfast throws the proven biochemistry of gluconeogenesis right out the window.

As a matter of fact, we are just fine without eating a meal, and when skipping a meal is done backed with some knowledge of how and why to do it properly, we can upgrade our bodily functions to their optimum potential. After all, really, the only thing science has ever proven about food is that calorie restriction leads to a longer life span.

Here again, I must acknowledge, there is nothing conceptually wrong with breakfast. It is not a terrible idea. However, when you look at the Standard American breakfast, it is an outright horrible idea. The SAD breakfast is the epitome of the ultra-processed, highly palatable, high sugar, low-nutrient junk food. Just look at the sugar content and ingredient list of one of your favorite cereals and you will wake up to this fact. If it is not a carbohydrate-based cereal, then it's a bagel, toast, pancakes, waffles, English muffin, fruit smoothie, biscuit, breakfast burrito, the list goes on and on. These are all high-carbohydrate, sugar spikes first thing in the morning. Not to mention most of them are highly processed "not food" the body does not recognize as actual food. We have been told to set the stage with a sugar spike in our body for breakfast. Now we receive a drastic increase in blood sugar and therefore insulin, giving our body an excess of energy, which is entirely too much. What does the body do with the excess energy (i.e., glucose)? Well, that's easy. The body is beyond intelligent, so it stores it away in adipose tissue as reserve for when we may need it.

After the body works its magic with this highly inflammatory sugar storm and creates homeostasis again, the cells of the body start to become anxious, looking for their habitual fix. They need sugar! They are hungry! At least we think that feeling is hunger. So now we are on our way to a snack and guess what? All the so-called "healthy" protein bars are loaded with what? Yup, you guessed it, sugar, toxic oils and sick animal protein.

You can see the rollercoaster your body is going through trying to metabolize this SAD. This creates inflammation in the body, and inflammation in the body eventually turns into pain and disease of some sort.

Enter intermittent fasting. All this means is that we go without eating or at least spiking our blood sugar for 13-18 hours or more if your metabolism is adapted to it. There are a variety of ways to incorporate this into your life. The most common way is to skip breakfast, not eating from dinner the night before until around lunch the next day, depending on when you stopped eating dinner. If you stopped eating dinner at 8:00 p.m. the previous evening, and you are just starting and working on a 16-hour fast, then you would eat your first meal at around 12:00 noon the next day. If this seems too extreme, simple. Cut it back to where you feel comfortable, but make sure you start with at least a 13-hour window of not eating since this ensures you start to utilize your stored body fat for energy (gluconeogenesis).

There is a lot happening in the body when we eat. The concept here is to stop the lot happening and let the body get around to doing what it naturally does. We are either in an anabolic state or a catabolic state. When we are in a fed or anabolic state, we are producing the hormones in our body, particularly insulin, which signals the cells that we are fed. This high insulin state is what leads to us getting fat. Insulin is present to allow the sugar from our food to enter the cells of our body. But because our food is so sugar rich and nutrient poor, we have too much sugar (glucose) in the blood. Basically, the cells of our body will not take any more sugar (glucose) because they have plenty. So, they close their doors. The body still produces insulin as a result of the sugar bomb unloaded from our last meal or snack. You should understand now that this is how we gain weight.

When we are constantly in this fed state, we are always storing fat, not using it for energy. Most Americans today are living year after year in this anabolic fed state. Over time, these continually high insulin levels result in high blood pressure as insulin in the blood retains fluid making the pressure in the blood vessels rise, arthritis as insulin causes inflammation in the joints, and diabetes as the cell stops responding to insulin because it is overburdened with glucose (sugar).

During the 16 hours of no food, our body first uses up the constituents of food from our previous meals. Next it burns through the glycogen stores in our liver. This is all a very intelligent design to keep our blood sugar levels stable. Once the glycogen stores have been used and after the 12-hour mark of fasting, our body switches over to a catabolic state in which our body uses its fat stores for fuel. This means we are now burning our stored fat for fuel. The hormonal signature of our body shifts, and now glucagon is the main hormone present. Glucagon catalyzes the mobilization of fat stores, which allows them to breakdown and turn into glucose or sugar. This allows our blood sugar to remain at an even level and keep from dropping. Glucagon also causes more blood flow to our heart, brain and muscles. Glucagon and the series of events happening in the catabolic state reduce inflammation throughout the body. Fat cells also eliminate stored toxins. We become more alert, focused and sharp as the increased blood flow to the brain wakes us up.

So much of what we do daily is wrapped up in our food routines—what we are going to eat, if we are eating the right thing, etc. Intermittent fasting gives us an opportunity to listen to our gut's innate intelligence as it is not having to focus on its contents of breakfast. Besides this, our body is able to regain its innate capacity to heal and regenerate when we are not eating by reducing the toxic stress put on it through the SAD. Even if you are eating a perfectly healthy diet, this food is still contaminated with toxins, and fasting gives your body time to reset and renew. Fasting has been used for thousands of years by almost all cultures to gain a greater spiritual connection. This should now make sense as when the gut goes into restoration mode, not having an excess of food contents, it can connect with the rest of the other energy centers of the body and elevate its now available energy to the heart and more.

Stepping into the unknown and skipping a meal can be a very scary thing. It was for me. We have conditioned our body to eat three meals a day ever since we can remember. This a deeply ingrained habit. Go easy on yourself and make sure you feel confident in your decision to do it. But remember on the other side of the unknown is the magic. Intermittent fasting is a huge step in taking your power back. It is your body. It is your life, and you get to decide.

Here are a few suggestions to help you through this life changing technique and reduce the fear of the unknown.

1.  Supplement MCT (Medium Chain Triglyceride) Oil during your fast. This is a fat derived from coconut oil, palm kernel oil, and dairy products. Coconut oil has the highest percentage in its fat profile with 15% being medium-chain triglycerides. MCT oil has amazing medicinal properties. It is colorless, odorless and tasteless. When this oil is eaten during a fast, it

does not affect the blood sugar, keeping your body in homeostasis. It also suppresses hunger while producing an energy component for our brain and body called ketones. After passing through the stomach, it is absorbed into the villi of the shag carpet lining of the intestinal wall. Because of its medium chain size, it is absorbed via the capillaries of the intestines and sent directly to the liver via the hepatic portal vein. Only small- and medium-chain triglycerides are absorbed by the portal vein because of their important properties which the body can use for fuel. All other fats are packaged into a molecule called a chylomicron and digested into the lymph system, which also has connections in the villi of the submucosa membrane. The lymphatic system is our safety net where all the toxic chemicals from our food and environment go to be dealt with by our immune system. The portal vein has evolved to be the extractor of the most useful nutrients for our body's health. The chain length of this medium-chain fat is what the portal vein is after as it accepts fatty acids of only 10-carbon chain lengths or less and sends them directly to the liver without having to go through the entire digestive process. These fats have no wait time like they would if they were digested through the typical digestion process, being sorted and checked by our immune system. Instead, after going straight to the liver, they are quickly converted into ketones. Ketones are extremely important molecules distributed throughout the body, the brain and heart to be used for energy. An important note on purchasing MCT oil. Make sure to buy a product that is labeled as a C6, C8 or C10 medium-chain triglyceride. These are Caproic, Caprylic and Capric saturated fatty acids, respectively. The number denotes the carbon chain length as the C denotes the carbon molecule. Be sure not to use C12 (Lauric Acid) as this fatty acid's carbon chain is too long to be sent through the Hepatic Portal Vein. MCT manufacturers use C12 (lauric acid) in combination with C8 in the processing of the oil to make more profit as C12 is more abundant in the coconut oil.

2.  Drink bulletproof coffee in the morning during your fast by combining a cup of coffee, 1-2 tablespoons of grass-fed butter or ghee and 1 teaspoon of MCT oil in a blender and blend together for 30 seconds. You can gradually increase the MCT oil amount as you feel your stomach can handle it. It is best to use a Blendtec, Vitamix or a blender with a glass jar as the hot contents can damage other blenders. If you enjoy coffee, this invention gives you an amazingly creamy cup of goodness. This will allow you to reap all the benefits of fasting but not have the hunger pangs that can come when not being used to skipping breakfast. This coffee and fat do not spike insulin levels and give your body the benefit of short-chain fatty acids from butter and MCTs. I recommend using the highest quality ingredients like grass-fed unsalted butter (Kerrygold is the most widely available) and high quality MCT oil. Bulletproof does it right with their products, although there are many other products on the market just as honest. It is important to use coffee of the highest quality and even tested for mold toxins that are present in much of the conventional coffee because it sits in large bags in humid warehouses where mold can easily grow.

3. If you do not like coffee, supplement coconut oil or MCT oil to boost fat burning metabolism. Just a warning—too much MCT (start with a teaspoon) can cause diarrhea. A spoonful of coconut oil should do the trick. MCT is a fat derived from coconuts, so there is MCT naturally occurring in coconut oil.

## Circadian Rhythms

Circadian rhythms are the rhythms of synchronizations in our body that each organ and hormone-producing glands (energy centers) operate within. The sleep and wake cycle is the most well-known circadian rhythm, but scientists are discovering a whole communication network within these energetic rhythms throughout our entire body. These rhythms are utilized for our tissues, organs and glands to regenerate, repair and reset.

What they are discovering is that time-restricted feeding (this is just another name for intermittent fasting) plays a primary role in the realignment of the body's circadian rhythms. It makes sense as we now know the rollercoaster the entire body goes through when eating the SAD is throwing the body's rhythms way out of whack. By simply eating your food within a window of let us say 12:00 noon to 7:00 p.m., your body is able to reset, repair and regenerate throughout the fasting period. Thus, allowing the rhythms to come back to their synchronization and optimizing our health.

Sleep is a non-negotiable. We must have it. And it is well known that shift workers are at much higher risk for developing disease in their body. This is clearly obvious as their circadian rhythms are imbalanced from being awake at night and sleeping during the day, leading to the cascade of disease in the body. Interesting, though most of us are doing some of the same amount of disruption with our sleeping habits. One of the main causes of this is blue light.

Blue light stimulates our pineal gland to trick our mind into believing it is day. When the sun goes down, our pineal gland naturally starts to increase melatonin, signaling our body to start winding down for bed. In today's world, though, few folks are getting ready for bed right after sundown. This is due to our wildly busy lives with crazy schedules and not enough time. When the sun goes down, many of us are finally able to relax and watch TV or catch up with our loved ones. All the lights in our house are on, we are watching TV, or we are on our phones. All this is emitting blue light, signaling our brain it is still day time. We are continuing the over-stimulation of our brain with the programming of the TV shows and the addiction to social media, thus further disrupting our circadian rhythms.

There is nothing wrong with staying up when it is dark. In fact, some do their best work after the sun goes down. However, there are some actions you can take to reconnect your circadian rhythms back online after the sun goes down.

1. Wear blue-light blocking glasses. If you like to watch TV or work on the computer at night, this is a great option.

2. Set the night shift mode on your phone to turn on at sunset and turn off at sunrise.

3. Turn off lights when the sun goes down or at least two hours before bed.

4. Use amber lightbulbs for lighting, like pink Himalayan salt lamps, orange or amber night lights or even amber light bulbs.

5. Install Flux on your computer. Flux is a free software that will change the light emitted from your computer screen to an amber color at night.

6. Meditate before bed. There is nothing more powerful than meditation when it comes to your circadian rhythms. As you fully relax and let go of the analytical mind, the body is able to work its magic and recalibrate. For extra benefit, meditating both in the morning right when you wake and at night can regenerate the cadence of serotonin and melatonin production, setting the stage for wakefulness and sleep, realigning your circadian rhythms. Not to mention, when you meditate before bed you are calming the analytical mind to slow down and allow for falling asleep.

The sleep/wake circadian rhythm is set in the morning when the sun rises. One very powerful tool you can do provides a double bonus when intermittent fasting. Get outside during or right after sunrise. Go on a walk, work in the garden, take the dog out or even just go check the mailbox. By doing this, you are telling your brain and body that it is day. The sunlight ramps up the serotonin hormone, which is the waking hormone. This will help set the clock for the day so that when the sun goes down that evening, melatonin production is in better rhythm. This, combined with fasting, is a great tool to synchronize your body's circadian rhythms.

## Smart Dollars

The way you buy is the most important thing you can do for your health, your family's health, and the future of our planet. Industrialized capitalization has scorched our earth of its natural resources. Depleting the life from our soil, chopping down crucial ecosystems of rain forest, dirtying the water we drink, fishing our fish into extinction, and polluting the air we breathe, we have taken our yearning for profit and power a bit too far. There is a change in the air. Millions of people around the world are waking up to what we are doing to our earth. We are connecting the dots of how the massive industrialized control over agriculture, pharmaceuticals, natural resources, etc. is contributing to our stressed out, chronically diseased bodies.

If you are like me, you may want to find the most beautiful plot of land with a crystal-clear stream flowing gracefully through it, never being touched by man, and make it your own self-sustaining farm. However, families, health insurance, mortgages, and jobs have led us down a different life path. What the heck can we do to change the world?

Practice emotional intelligence (Section Two) and learn to become aware of what the external factors in our world are doing to our emotions. Practice the refractory period to get back to the emotion of the dream future you have created. Stay in that energy throughout the day pausing to make sure you get back to it.

Stop buying the products of those of the very few who control the seed, agriculture and dairy industries.

Buy local. Find the nearest farmers market, preferably organic and ask questions. Buy what you feel is the most ethically sourced, freshest picked, nutrient dense products that you know. Purchase with love. Knowing that you are creating a circle of health for you, them, the animal, the soil and the earth. Feel gratitude to give your hard-earned dollar to the local farmer to generate abundance for both wealth and health.

Start your own garden. Start small and plant some organic seeds. Tend to them, love them and watch them grow. There is no better way to appreciate food than by growing it yourself.

Buy from the companies that do it right. Research the efficacy of the company claiming an organic, sustainable product. Feel it in your heart that this company is legit. When you purchase their product, embrace how good it feels to be supporting their efforts to make this world a better place.

I know these above-mentioned steps may seem very menial, but this is where change has to start. A grassroots effort is what it takes to truly make a difference. By supporting a more logical, common sense and sustainable practice, the masses will soon realize there is a better way. No protests needed, just pure ingenuity of a much more justifiable method. The scales will tip.

By gaining this knowledge, you are creating a new level of understanding. You have increased your awareness, and that creates a higher consciousness to make better decisions. The healing power of food is another tool you now can utilize and epigenetically create your healthiest self. As we choose to eat the most whole, real foods we can find, we begin to create diverse and healthy soil in our gut (microbiome), just as diversifying crop rotation creates a healthier soil. Choosing high-quality food has a much higher and potential epigenetic signal to our bodies. This signaling creates a higher vibration in all our cells and tissues, creating a higher vibration within and all around us. When you are vibrating at this higher frequency and feel better than you ever have, now you start to see feedback in your life. Healthier skin, weight loss, increased muscle tone, decreased pain, laser sharp focus, etc.

# Conclusion – Wholeness

Emotional Intelligence is integrated into the curriculum at my daughter's school. I was overjoyed knowing my daughter and the rest of the young impressionable children would be learning something so essential to create a better world. One of my daughter's lessons in her first-grade class was to learn what it means to fill someone else's bucket. Again, I was thrilled to hear from her teacher through her weekly email updates that the students were going to learn about what it feels like to make others feel good. In essence, they were going to learn to give.

When we are balanced in our emotional awareness, and we better understand where our attention and energy are being directed, then when we give, we receive. For giving is receiving. It is the circle of life. Here is how I distinguish it.

We wake up to the fact that we are the creators of what we desire in our life, and then we set our intention on manifesting it. This becomes our purpose and passion. When our creation manifests in our three-dimensional world, we are awe inspired that it actually happened, and we know we created it. Guess what we do? Well, because we feel so whole and complete knowing we have created it, we cannot help but share this feeling of love. So, we give our gifts of love to others. Those gifts which we have created. We become selfless because we realize we are the creator of our desire, and there is no lack in the inexhaustible field of energy all around us. There is only abundance. This means we can create from scratch again. This giving then comes back to us in a number of ways. One, because it feels so darn good to give, and we reap the rewards in our physical body epigenetically and psychoneuroimmunologically. This results in an overall increase of energy. Two, because we are living in an elevated state, we match vibrationally with potentials in the field, and sure enough amazing synchronicities, serendipities and new opportunities show up in our physical reality. Whoa! Awe inspired! Give! Share! And then it comes back. This completes the circle again and again. Wholeness.

So after thinking about the email I received from my daughter's first grade teacher, it dawned on me that if my daughter is only learning to fill someone else's bucket without learning how to fill her own, she is missing out on one of life's most important lessons. I realized I must teach her what it means to fill her own bucket in order to have enough to give to others in whatever shape or form that may be. I became inspired to teach her how this works. Of course, I wanted her to learn the importance of giving, but without learning how to again regenerate what we give, we can begin to crave the giving. Or we can develop a habit of avoiding our own needs just to feel the rush of giving to others. This would be like a heart that only pumps out oxygenated blood without receiving the deoxygenated blood back to be replenished. It is not a complete system, and problems will ensue.

I explained it to her like this. Imagine that you live next to a beautiful stream that flows abundantly. This stream allows you to always have a full bucket of water. Now imagine you have a friend at school that does not have access to the stream like you do. She has a bucket too, but her bucket only has a bit of water. Water she may have left over from what her mom or dad gave her or what she got at school. Either way, her bucket is not all the way full. So being kind and generous like you were taught to be, you give her as much as she needs to fill her bucket back to the top. Now your water is lower, but her bucket is full, and you feel amazing after giving what you had to her.

(Here is the part that was missing.) I asked her, "So what are you going to do to fill your bucket back up?"

Without hesitation, she said, "Refill it again."

She nailed it! Of course, she did. It is totally obvious. I then explained to her we must fill our bucket back up with our own power. If we intend to give all that we have, in whatever context that may be, we must have a full bucket. Otherwise, our bucket will run dry, and we will have nothing left to sustain ourselves.

To fill our own bucket is to love ourselves. In order to love others with all our hearts, we must first love ourselves. The more we have of it for ourselves, the more we can give to others. Just as the flight attendant instructs in the pre-flight announcements, in case of an emergency landing and oxygen masks are deployed, you must first put the oxygen mask on yourself before helping any small children. For if you do not have oxygen, you cannot help the child in need. The same thing goes for the bucket analogy. If you want water to give, you must come home and fill your bucket again and again with the abundant supply within and all around us. This is common sense. It is so simple, and we all know it innately, yet we are so easily tricked into separation from it. The question is, can you be greater than your environment and practice this day in and day out?

In the analogy I taught my daughter, the abundantly flowing stream is the infinite intelligence of the quantum field constantly around us and within us, waiting for us to tap into. It loves us more than we can imagine. Despite and without any conditions in our external world. When we learn to sustain this almost indescribable feeling that feels so familiar, we learn how to become aware of when we are in that state and when we are not. The state of this high vibration of love is who we really are. It is our natural state. As we practice and tend to the generation of this state, we feel this indescribable love grow. Just as the mighty oak tree grows from a tiny acorn. The practice of cultivating this love in our mind and body generates a feeling of wholeness inside us. And just as the oak grows slowly but surely, the love inside our cells does too. The growth of this intentionally created love generates the fabric of our DNA to rewrite our gene expression. This is like a magical key that unlocks an unbreakable lock on a hidden treasure chest. This is how we unleash our unlimited potential in every cell of our body. This book has given you the key you now have to practice.

### DO THE WORK!

When something is whole, there is nothing missing. The thing is complete. It already has everything. We are whole. We already have all we are looking for. When we feel whole and embody this state, we appreciate that we already have whatever it is we are looking for. Whilst living in lower states below the awareness of wholeness, we are fooled into thinking that whatever we are searching for to make us healthy, happy or wealthy is a thing. We are tricked into believing it will come from something separate from us. But this is only an illusion. When we can comprehend and understand neurologically that we are already whole, we start to realize we do not need anything from the outside world. We actually comprehend that we are everything. We are one. Singular. When we are in the state of oneness or wholeness, our body now receives this new neurological order via the neuropeptides it releases. And neuropeptides signal the cell to unlock the magic in the DNA.

In the state of wholeness, oneness or singularity, there is no separation. We are not separate from that which we are seeking because we already are it. For it is us and we are it; therefore, it cannot be separate from us. Yet again, we will be pulled back into our old programs, and this will time and time again fool us into separation because of the illusion of the third dimension that we are currently living in. This is where the work comes in. We must remember because we have practiced so many times how to generate the indescribable feeling of wholeness and then get right back to that feeling. Wholeness creates this most amazing feeling of indescribable love. Again, we understand that no person, nothing, no place or no time is separate from us in the quantum reality. Now we are back into coherence and redirect our attention, energy and innate healing power back into ourselves.

As we learn to live our life not separate from anything, we begin to have compassion for everyone, everything and every place on this earth because we are it. We realize if we judge or hate another, we are only judging and hating ourselves. We would never want to hurt our mother earth because she is us. We take off our suit of armor and sheath our sword, becoming humble. We surrender to a process so much bigger than we are that is unfolding before us. We turn our own demons into allies because we know they are all one. Compassion fills our heart with more love, and we now understand what those feelings create chemically, hormonally and genetically in our body. Why would we not want to give ourselves this inherent gift that is already built in? This is our health! We can heal because we create the program to do so.

# Further Reading

*The Bulletproof Diet* by Dave Asprey

*Biology of Belief* by Bruce Lipton

*Why Zebras Don't Get Ulcers* by Robert M. Sapolsky

*The Power of Eight* by Lynn McTaggert

*The Science of Self Empowerment* by Gregg Braden

*Grow a New Body* by Alberto Villoldo

*Stealing Fire* by Steven Kolter, Jamie Wheal

*Discovering Your Soul Signature* by Panache Desai

*The Four Agreement* by don Miguel Ruiz

*The Energy Codes* by Sue Morter

*Living in The Heart* by Drunvalo Melchizedek

*Gut* by Giulia Enders

*Evolve Your Brain* by Joe Dispenza

*You Are the Placebo* by Joe Dispenza

*Breaking the Habit of Being Yourself* by Joe Dispenza

*Becoming Supernatural* by Joe Dispenza

*Meta Human* by Deepak Chopra

*The Craving Mind* by Judson Brewer

*Wired to Eat* by Robb Wolf

*Genius Foods* by Max Lugavere and Paul Grewal

*Food: What the Heck Should I Eat* by Mark Hyman

*The Longevity Diet* by Valter Longo

*Human Heart, Cosmic Heart* by Thomas Cowan

*The Hungry Brain: Outsmarting the Instincts That Make Us Overeat* by Stephan J. Guyenet

*The Power of Eight* by Lynne McTaggart

*Believe in People: Bottom-Up Solutions For a Top-Down World* by Charles Kock, Steve Carlson

*The Wim Hof Method: Activate Your Full Human Potential* by Wim Hof

*Regenerate: Unlocking Your Body's Radical Resilience Through the New Biology* by Sayer Ji

*The Plant Paradox: The Hidden Dangers in Healthy Foods That Cause Disease* by Steven R. Gundry

# Reference

1. Sauver, JL et al. "Why patients visit their doctors: Assessing the most prevalent conditions in a defined American population." Mayo Clinic Proceedings, Volume 88, Issue 1, 56–67.

2. Cherkin, Daniel C. PhD; Deyo, Richard A. MD, MPH; Loeser, John D. MD; Bush, Terry PhD; Waddell, Gordon BSc, MD, FRCS "An International Comparison of Back Surgery Rates" Spine. June 1, 1994 - Volume 19 - Issue 11 - p 1201-1206. https://insights.ovid.com/crossref?an=00007632-199405310-00001

3. Losina E, Thornhill TS, Rome BN, Wright J, Katz JN. "The dramatic increase in total knee replacement utilization rates in the United States cannot be fully explained by growth in population size and the obesity epidemic" J Bone Joint Surg Am. February 1, 2012; 94(3):201-207. doi:10.2106/JBJS.J.01958. https://www.ncbi.nlm.nih.gov/pmc/articles/PMC3262184/

4. Lipton, Bruce. The Biology of Belief. Carlsbad: Hay House, Inc., 2015. Print

5. Meador, C K. "Hex death: voodoo magic or persuasion?" South Med J 1992; 85; 244–247.

6. Dispenza, Joe. Breaking the Habit of Being Yourself. Carlsbad: Hay House, Inc. 2012. Print

7. Cowan, Thomas. Human Heart Cosmic Heart. White River Junction: Chelsea Green Publishing. 2016. Print

8. Lancaster University. "Global study reveals time running out for many soils, but conservation measures can help." ScienceDaily. ScienceDaily, 14 September 2020. https://www.sciencedaily.com/releases/2020/09/200914115905.htm

9. Asprey, D. (can't find the date). "Glyphosate: Why Eating Organic Really Does Matter." Asprey, Dave. https://daveasprey.com/glyphosate-why-eating-organic-really-does-matter/

10. Fasano A, Sapone A, Zevallos V, Schuppan D. "Nonceliac gluten sensitivity." Gastroenterology. 2015 May;148(6):1195-204. doi: 10.1053/j.gastro.2014.12.049. Epub 2015 Jan 9. PMID: 25583468.

11. University of Colorado Denver. (2013, February 19). "Diet of resistant starch helps the body resist colorectal cancer." ScienceDaily. Retrieved March 24, 2021 from www.sciencedaily.com/releases/2013/02/130219140716.htm

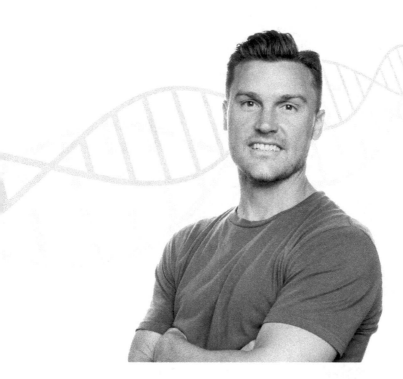

# About the Author

Cason has spent the last 10 years working as a Physical Therapist Assistant and now a Holistic Health Coach. After setting records as a college athlete, Cason found himself 70 pounds overweight, loaded with chronic pain. Cason was working his dream job relieving his patient's pain as a PTA, however he found himself unable to heal his own ailments.

Stressed, irritable and overweight he found that eating real whole food, applying movement strategies and practicing meditation, were the key to his healing. Since then Cason has never looked back. Being driven by the belief that every human being is capable of healing all dis-ease, Cason's passion is to inspire others to live in this mindset of unlimited potential.

Cason is the proud husband and father to Chancey and Cutler.